Doctor, What Should I Eat?

The Best Treatment

Symptoms

Modern Prevention

Second Opinion

The Complete Medical Exam

*The Electrocardiogram and
Chest X-ray in Diseases
of the Heart*

DR. ROSENFELD'S
GUIDE TO
ALTERNATIVE
MEDICINE

DR. ROSENFELD'S GUIDE TO ALTERNATIVE MEDICINE

❖ ❖ ❖

What Works, What Doesn't—
and What's Right for You

ISADORE ROSENFELD, M.D.

RANDOM HOUSE

NEW YORK

Author's Note

Nothing in this book can replace the services of a trained physician. I have written it to help you make more informed choices for your health care and to help you work more effectively with your physician. It is particularly important in the realm of alternative medicine, in which there are still so many unknowns, to keep your physician informed if you're considering any of the alternative therapies described in this book.

Grateful acknowledgment is made to the following for permission to reprint previously published material:

University of Texas–Houston: Yoga instruction from the January 1996 *Lifetime Health Letter.* Reprinted by permission of the University of Texas–Houston.

Journal of Alternative and Complementary Medicine: Excerpt from article from Vol. 2, 1996, pp. 211–248. Reprinted by permission of *Journal of Alternative and Complementary Medicine.*

Library of Congress Cataloging-in-Publication Data
Rosenfeld, Isadore.
Dr. Rosenfeld's guide to alternative medicine : what works, what doesn't—and what's right for you / Isadore Rosenfeld.
p.   cm.
Includes index.
ISBN 0-679-42817-8
1. Alternative medicine—Popular works.   I. Title.
R733.R675   1997
615.5—dc20   96-30558

Random House website address: http://www.randomhouse.com/
Printed in the United States of America on acid-free paper
2 4 6 8 9 7 5 3
First Edition

*For my wife, children, and grandchildren
(welcome aboard, Jesse Alexander),
who are a greater source of health and
happiness to me than any medicine—
conventional or alternative*

ACKNOWLEDGMENTS

In all of my previous books, I have dedicated pages to thanking the many M.D.s, nutritionists, and other members of the medical community who were kind enough to review my manuscript. However, given the often contentious debate over alternative medicine, I have deliberately chosen not to send the finished manuscript of this book for formal review to any conventional or alternative practitioners, although I did show chapters informally to experts in both camps. I feared that conventional doctors would find the content too permissive, while alternative practitioners would consider it too critical. Truth is never universally popular. My conclusions and recommendations are based on extensive review of the existing scientific evidence and the literature about alternative medicine, on conversations with patients, and on my own personal experience. With this book I hope to help bridge the gap between the two communities, because I believe that it is with their union that we will find our best options for health care.

As usual, thanks to my editor, Betsy Rapoport, whose inspired editing warrants an N.D. and/or an M.D.

CONTENTS

Contents

Contents

INTRODUCTION
Times Are Changing!

Why are millions of Americans, especially those who are better educated, spending billions of dollars every year on a wide variety of "alternative," "complementary," or "holistic" therapies such as herbs, acupuncture, and meditation? Why are they either abandoning treatments recommended by their regular doctors or supplementing prescribed therapies with some other regimen that much of the medical "establishment" rejects or ridicules? And why are they doing so in view of the stunning achievements of the medical establishment? Just think. Using the scientific method, doctors have made it possible to bypass your coronary arteries; to change your heart valves; and to repair or replace your heart, liver, and kidneys and most of your joints. Cosmetic surgeons can leave you looking half your age. Your genes can be manipulated, and several inherited diseases can be prevented or cured. There are powerful new antibiotics to eradicate infections that used to kill. There are drugs to control pain, restore your sex drive, open the airways to your lungs, shrink your enlarged prostate, melt your gallstones, and promptly end migraine attacks. There are machines to shatter your kidney stones and regulate your heart rhythm. There are ways to remove your gallstones, appendix, ovaries, and other prized possessions without even cutting you open. Virtually invisible hearing aids can restore your lost hearing; you are able to read again the very next morning after your cataracts have been removed. So why the rush to explore radically different avenues of treatment?

The growing popularity of alternative medicine, despite all the accomplishments of medical science in this century, is the direct result of the many questions relating to health, well-being, and survival that remain unanswered. In the words of one great physician, Sir William Osler, "Medicine is a science of uncertainty and an art of probability." Yes, we *are* living longer and better, thanks to antibiotics, safer anesthetics, improved surgical techniques, and innovative technical devices. But this longer life span has, at the same time, left us vulnerable to many degenerative diseases that cripple and kill. We continue to suffer and die from cancer, rheumatoid arthritis, Parkinson's disease, multiple sclerosis, Alzheimer's disease, AIDS, and emphysema. There is no way to stop arteries from clogging, cataracts from forming, prostates from enlarging, migraines from starting, or kidneys and livers from failing. These ailments can sometimes be slowed but rarely prevented or cured. Worse, many of our "best available" treatments are ineffective and end up only prolonging the agony of death.

So the sick and vulnerable are hungry for other options, of which the most accessible, understandable, and appealing to the layperson is alternative medicine. Healthy people are also exploring, or at least considering, some form of alternative medicine because of the perception that following some of its basic tenets can help prevent disease *before* it starts—not always the primary goal of conventional medicine.

Another reason alternative medicine is gaining credibility is because the established medical profession is losing credibility—in part because doctors always seem to be changing their minds. Theories and practices that were presented as sacrosanct, indisputable, and inviolable often turn out to be harmful in the long run. Here are just a few examples of how conventional medicine has reversed its position on some important theories and practices:

- Thirty years ago, following a heart attack, the rule was six weeks of complete bed rest—no phone calls, few visitors, and only a bedpan for diversion. In those days, any doctor who permitted such a patient to sit up at the edge of the bed after only one or two days, or sent him or her home in a week, as I do today, would have been severely criticized and would probably have lost his or her hospital privileges.
- In the mid 1970s, when Nathan Pritikin theorized that a low-fat, low-cholesterol diet, along with exercise, could reduce the incidence of heart disease, he was ridiculed by most doctors. That's because he was only a "Mr." and not an M.D. Twenty-five years later, those who were his most vocal detractors then are now practicing what he preached.
- Giving a nitroglycerin tablet under the tongue to relieve chest pain during an acute heart attack was also a major no-no. Today, doctors administer nitroglycerin to heart attack victims immediately—and intravenously!
- Not so long ago, if you had gallstones you were whisked into a hospital and had your gallbladder taken out without delay, even if you were symptom-free. Today, your doctor will probably advise against such surgery unless and until you develop symptoms.

• Think of all the lives that might have been lost had we scoffed at, and not tested, the "ridiculous" idea that an aspirin a day helps prevent strokes and heart attacks.

Small wonder, then, that there is growing conviction that despite its past and ongoing "miracles," the medical establishment is not infallible and should take a hard look at some fresh and different concepts, philosophies, and approaches to the prevention and treatment of disease.

Why have most doctors refused to do so? I can assure you that it's not because of any conspiracy to withhold cures and breakthroughs from the American people. All those books and magazine articles "exposing" the many "secrets your doctor won't tell you because they threaten his income" are paranoid hogwash. One reason for this reluctance is a fear that legitimizing alternative approaches may encourage patients to abandon treatments with a proven track record. That's why some doctors feel more comfortable with the term "complementary medicine," which implies a merger of "conventional" and "unconventional" techniques—rather than the wholesale disavowal of established therapies. Also, M.D.s are trained to look at facts, not act on rumors. The Hippocratic oath requires them to "first, do no harm," to be cautious and careful in choosing any treatment, and to be convinced that it has a reasonable chance of success. The fact remains that much of alternative medicine has *not* been subjected to the rigorous scientific scrutiny high medical standards demand.

But the gap between "conventional" and "unconventional" practitioners is narrowing, as more and more doctors (and patients) realize that the "other" medicine can no longer be ignored, that *any* rational and promising approach must be evaluated impartially and scientifically. One of the main reasons for this attitude, in addition to societal pressure, is that newer diagnostic techniques, and the appreciation of the tie between the brain (where emotion is generated) and the immune system (whose strength and integrity determine vulnerability and resistance to disease), have resulted in a better understanding of how some forms of alternative medicine may be effective.

Alternative medicine has one foot out of the closet; its "brown-paper wrapper" has been torn away. Patients with cancer, especially those who have been "written off," are trying hypnosis or acupuncture to control their pain, meditating, engaging in spiritual therapy, or experimenting with special diets. Chances are that if you have chronic backaches, your doctor may advise you to see a chiropractor or acupuncturist, or to try a relaxation technique or a "bodyworks" treatment. If you have chronic insomnia, don't be surprised if your doctor first suggests chamomile tea or valerian at bedtime, before writing a prescription for a sleeping pill. And should you muster the courage to ask about chelation, royal jelly, or coffee enemas, while you will probably be told they're worthless, your doctor will at least discuss them with you.

Even the National Institutes of Health, the very embodiment of the medical establishment, is expressing interest in some unorthodox therapies. At last count, its recently formed Office of Alternative Medicine and various other agencies of the federal government were spending more than $23 million a year to evaluate such diverse approaches as acupuncture for drug abuse, anti-HIV activity in plant compounds, and the efficacy of chiropractic. Several health insurance companies, such as American Western Life Insurance, Mutual of Omaha, a few Blue Cross plans, and others—members of an industry not especially known for its compassion or generosity—are now reimbursing policyholders who participate in "wellness" plans that include the

Pritikin and Ornish programs for prevention of heart disease, as well as acupuncture, chiropractic, naturopathy, and techniques for relaxation and reduction of stress. And in 1997, the Oxford Health Plan began reimbursing for a wide variety of alternative therapies.

There has even been a softening toward "unconventional" medicine in academe. A Center for the Study of Alternative Medicine has been established by my friends Richard and Hinda Rosenthal at the medical school of Columbia University, offering elective courses for students, and seminars for interested health care professionals. More than a score of other medical schools have followed suit. Given its almost absolute authority with respect to what is "good" and "bad" in medical care, this new interest and flexibility on the part of "organized medicine" (by no means unanimous—there is still a core of diehards) is all the more remarkable. Establishment doctors are still demanding proof, as they should, but at least they're looking outside their own bailiwick.

In this book, I devote a separate chapter to each of the most widely used methods in alternative medicine. But before dealing with specifics, let me introduce you to the concept of "holism," which you will encounter throughout these pages, and, indeed, whenever alternative medicine is discussed. "Holistic" doctors say they differ from conventional physicians in these ways:

- They consider the mind and body to be a single entity.
- They believe that good health is a positive state, not merely the absence of disease, and that the patient must work to preserve it. Prevention, not treatment, is their first priority.
- They believe the body can often heal itself without medication.
- They look at the whole patient rather than any one organ or system. (How often have you heard yourself referred to

on the intercom in your doctor's office or emergency room as "the gallbladder," "the flu shot," or "the chest pain in room 3"?)

- They pay more attention to the impact of the total environment on bodily functions, delving more thoroughly into the kind of food you're eating, whether or not you smoke, how much you drink, how much you exercise, and how happy you are with your lot in life.

None of this is new, revolutionary, or unique to holism. Many establishment doctors share these same beliefs. This is how I practice medicine and what I teach my students. Hippocrates, the "father of medicine," wrote long ago that "it is more important to know the person that has the disease than the disease the person has." Years later, Jan Christiaan Smuts, better known as a prime minister of South Africa than as the famous biologist he was, formalized this attitude and called it "wholistic." Like Hippocrates, he emphasized that the whole is greater than the sum of its parts. The real difference between mainstream doctors and those who formally designate themselves as "holistic" is that the latter also employ a wide variety of controversial treatment methods, from psychic healing, herbs, and megavitamins to immune therapy, homeopathy, reflexology, and naturopathy.

A word of warning: Unfortunately, many quacks and hustlers who call themselves "alternative practitioners" deal in fraud and deceit, not alternative medicine. Because of the hype that inevitably accompanies any "different" approach, you can never be sure what's real and legitimate, what will work and what won't, and whether it's safe to abandon the "tried and true" therapy recommended by your own doctor. There's really no place to obtain that information. If you investigate a particular complementary technique, you'll usually find that it's passionately and uncritically endorsed by its proponents, and violently and equally uncritically condemned by its detractors. There is no middle ground, very few open minds, and lots of name-calling.

I wrote this book to show that there *is* a middle ground. I hope it will provide answers to your questions, and that after reading it, you will be able to distinguish those treatments that may be useful from those that are futile, fraudulent, or fraught with danger. As a practicing doctor and member of the academic and medical establishment, who has tried promising alternative treatments, I have reviewed and evaluated the field unencumbered by preconceptions. In my search for the truth, I have interviewed many patients, including those who have ventured into the realm of alternative therapy; I have had frank discussions with many of its practitioners; and I have studied the world literature looking for documentation of the effectiveness of the more widely used unconventional treatments. I didn't find much in the traditional scientific journals because, quite frankly, the establishment has never encouraged the use of alternative therapies or reported their results. What studies there were rarely documented the claims made for "complementary" techniques. On the other hand, those done by "unconventional" practitioners and published in their own organs, while full of enthusiasm, are usually short on data. Keep in mind, though, that just because something hasn't been scientifically tested doesn't necessarily mean it can't be effective. Many of these interventions have been tested in the laboratory of human experience—and have passed with flying colors.

Scientific papers are generally replete with tables, statistics, and formulas, which, however boring, usually do support or disprove a theory. By contrast, the theme in virtually every alternative report is that the body is great; that *natural* healing powers can be enhanced by a variety of therapies; and that one's emotional, mental, and spiritual state is very important in the prevention and treatment of "physical" disease—concepts that may well be valid but do not lend themselves to statistical analysis. Practitioners of alternative medicine aren't really concerned about theory or about the mechanisms by which something works; they're interested in results. Chinese practitioners consider it a waste of time, energy, and money to do a placebo-controlled, double-blind study on an herb they are convinced works after thousands of years of use. By the same token, most traditional doctors trained in the scientific method are hesitant to use or recommend any approach whose efficacy has not been proven to their satisfaction. In the following chapters, we will see if and when this position is justified.

DR. ROSENFELD'S GUIDE TO ALTERNATIVE MEDICINE

THE LURE OF THE CURE

Because Hope Springs Eternal

The hype, hoopla, and reckless claims that accompany so much of alternative medicine make it hard to appraise it objectively. Just look at the ads for some of these therapies. They promise a cure for virtually every imaginable symptom and disease—overweight, fat thighs, heart attack, stroke, zero libido or poor sexual performance, arthritis, and even cancer. "Experts" on radio and TV talk shows, often using cleverly disguised infomercials, try to seduce you with tales of their miraculous discoveries. You have been deliberately kept in the dark by "organized" medicine for its own selfish purposes! Unfortunately, there are many to whom such nonsense offers a glimmer of hope. Someone suffering from an incurable, debilitating, or terminal disease is an easy target for even the wildest and most improbable promise. To ignore it is to shut the door on hope. It's only human to wonder whether maybe, just maybe, there is something to such a claim, however preposterous. So, with nothing to lose, people sometimes take the bait. The following are true accounts of what happened to some who did.

The mother of a famous cancer specialist I know was dying of lung cancer that had spread to her bones and brain. Chemotherapy and radiation had failed. Her son knew that there was no hope. But while the doctor in him had written her off, the son contacted a cancer clinic overseas that had no status with the scientific community. None of its grandiose claims had ever been substantiated. Although as a doctor he had never referred any patients to that clinic, as a son he was unable to resist the lure of the cure when his mother's life was at stake. They set off for Europe together.

The personnel at the clinic were refreshingly upbeat. The despondent patient and her son became cautiously optimistic; and after a few days, the son began to feel optimistic even as a doctor. The treatment regimen contained neither drugs nor radiation, since maximal doses of both had already been given. The patient received a "special" diet as well as several powders and herbs in which she was said to be deficient. (At home, she had been permitted to eat whatever she wanted in order to stop her weight loss.) The program of "total care" also included "cleansing enemas," group therapy with other cancer patients, and meditation. These measures, together with a very positive attitude, left this woman full of hope and confidence—a far cry from the sense of doom and hopelessness she'd experienced at the scientific cancer center back home.

A few weeks later, in the middle of this regimen, my colleague's mother died peacefully in her sleep. Had her trip to the clinic—the travel, the expense, the hope—been worth it? By the objective standards of scientific medicine, the expedition was an exercise in futility. But science gives no points for the equanimity, the calm, and the contentment the patient and her family enjoyed. I can tell you that neither as son nor as doctor did my friend regret his decision to try this "unconventional" approach. I have never since asked him whether he now sends any of his patients to this particular facility. What's your guess?

In this case, there was nothing to lose from exploring uncharted seas because everything else had been tried—and had failed. But that's not always so, as is illustrated in the following account.

A twenty-three-year-old woman came to see me because she was worried about several enlarged but painless lymph glands in both armpits and in her neck. They felt suspicious, so I had them biopsied (a piece of tissue was removed and examined under the microscope). The diagnosis was Hodgkin's disease, a cancer of the lymph system that used to be fatal but now can almost always be cured. I arranged for her to see a cancer specialist, who suggested a combination of radiation and chemotherapy that he was confident would result in a cure. To my dismay, the patient rejected this therapy because she had been persuaded by her family and friends to choose "nature's way" rather than be "poisoned" by toxic X rays and drugs. For two years she followed a macrobiotic diet, was given coffee enemas regularly, and consumed a variety of herbs. By the time it became apparent that this approach would not cure her disease, it was too late to save her.

This young woman and her family ignored the mountain of evidence *proving* that Hodgkin's disease can be cured by conventional methods. Neither she nor her advisers had asked for any statistics about the regimen she chose to follow instead. Her decision to pursue an "alternative" route was based on a deadly combination of blind faith, ignorance, and the all-too-common dread of chemotherapy. She paid for that decision with her life.

A legendary Greek shipowner who died some years ago is another example of how the lure of a cure can be a fatal attraction. He suffered from myasthenia gravis, a disorder in which muscles, mainly in the head and chest, do not contract effectively. He had trouble chewing his food and could eat only a soft diet; he couldn't keep his eyes open without raising his eyelids with Scotch tape. He worried that one day the disease would involve the muscles of his chest and that he would be unable to breathe. In most cases of myasthenia gravis, symptoms can be controlled by medication; people with this disorder are usually able to lead normal lives. But this man did not respond to the standard therapy. We tried several new and experimental drugs and were finally able to minimize his symptoms with large doses of steroids.

His doctors were delighted with his long remission, but the patient himself was terrified that the medication would lose its effectiveness. At that point, he began hearing glowing testimonials from an assortment of royalty, movie stars, and some very rich people about a "miracle" pill called GH3, which was (and remains) popular in Europe. Its Romanian developers claimed that it conferred virtually eternal youth —not to mention a sex drive with no expiration date and a full head of hair. GH3, despite all the mystique surrounding it, is simply the local anesthetic procaine (its trade name in this country is Novocain) that your dentist uses. When taken by mouth, it dilates the superficial blood vessels of the face and scalp, causing a flush that creates the impression that it's "working."

This patient decided to try GH3. The doctor who prescribed it convinced him that he could now stop taking steroids. Tragically, the doctor was unaware that procaine worsens myasthenia gravis. Several weeks after starting the drug, the patient's chewing and swallowing began to deteriorate, and he was soon back to eating baby food and taping his eyelids. He stopped the GH3 and resumed the cortisone, but the second time around, he did not respond as well to it. He died a few months later from complications of emergency gallbladder surgery.

My reason for recounting this particular story is not primarily to denigrate GH3. Although its benefits have never been proven to the satisfaction of the scientific community anywhere in the world, some of my own patients (though none with myasthenia gravis!) continue to take it without ill effect, and they insist that it makes them feel better. The importance of this case is that it illustrates how dangerous it can be to abandon an effective treatment in favor of *any* therapy, alternative or conventional, that has not been tested and shown to work.

Another patient, a woman of forty-eight, developed a hard lump on the right side of her neck. Biopsy revealed it to be a cancer that had originated in and spread from the base of the tongue. Her oncologist agreed that radiating her mouth and throat offered the best chance of cure, and that she would require some forty treatments. Unfortunately, X-ray therapy often burns the delicate tissues of the mouth, making eating painful, swallowing difficult, the tongue sore and swollen, and the teeth loose. When I forewarned the patient about all these possible complications, she consulted a specialist in alternative medicine. He advised her to have the radiation but to gargle with sesame oil before and after each session. The radiologist, the oncologist, and I were amused by this simplistic suggestion, but we did not object to it, because it could do no harm—and we had nothing better to offer.

Our patient began the combined X-ray therapy and sesame oil routine. To our astonishment, her mouth never became red and blistered, her tongue did not swell, she lost none of her teeth, and her ability to swallow remained intact! In follow-up exams, her oncologist reported to me that her mouth was "remarkably well hydrated with excellent saliva production, and she states that her taste is almost completely normal." In another chart note, he adds, "I have asked her to document in writing for us what substances, agents, and homeopathic drugs she used during her radiation therapy *in hopes that it might benefit other patients*. She clearly was extraordinarily positive throughout the course of the treatment, which was obviously to her great benefit."

None of the doctors involved in this case had ever seen anyone tolerate so much radiation so well. Although I can't be sure, I believe that it was the sesame oil that did the trick! In my view, this is an example of how patients can benefit when conventional and alternative practitioners work together to provide them with the best of both worlds.

If you are in the throes of a terminal disease such as cancer or AIDS, or you have a chronic condition that has caused more suffering than you can bear, your doctor *must* do the following: (1) Make absolutely certain that the diagnosis is correct, no matter how many "second opinions" it takes. (2) Investigate and try every treatment that has proven to be effective in cases like yours; or, if an experimental drug or treatment is available, make sure that it is safe and has a sound theoretical rationale before giving it to you. (3) Finally, if your disease has not responded to whatever is available, provide you with all the compassion and all the medication necessary to ensure your dignity and comfort.

But when all these obligations have been fulfilled, and nothing more can be done, *you* must assume responsibility for your own health and survival. Never lose hope. History is full of miracles. In practical terms, this means exploring alternatives, including those that happen to be outside your doctor's area of expertise. Your objective should be both to live longer and to enjoy the best possible quality of life. However, don't jump from the frying pan into the fire. Before trying any alternative, you and your doctor should investigate its track record as thoroughly as you can to make sure it won't make matters worse. Work with your doctor to document any effect—good or bad—of the proposed therapy.

❖ 2 ❖

THE PLACEBO RESPONSE

Are You and Your Doctor Blind?

Please don't just skim this chapter. Read it very carefully, because it will help you understand the heart of the controversy between alternative and conventional health practitioners. It explains why you need to view with caution every anecdotal account of a cure, however dramatic.

Several years ago, members of the cardiology department at our hospital were asked by a pharmaceutical company to evaluate a new drug for the treatment of angina pectoris, the chest pain or pressure induced by physical exertion or emotional stress in people with coronary artery disease. We selected fifty patients with this condition for the study. They were to be given two sets of pills, one active, and the other "placebo"—a blank. The active pill and the placebo were completely indistinguishable from each other in appearance, texture, taste, and smell. The tablets were to be switched every two weeks over a two-month period. We told the patients that we were testing a new and promising drug for angina, but did not inform them that half the time they would be taking "dummy" pills. (I'm not sure it's right to withhold such information, and were I doing this study today, I would disclose use of the placebo.) The subjects continued to take their regular antianginal medications, because it is dangerous and unethical to replace an agent that works with either a test drug of unproven efficacy or a placebo. None of the doctors knew which preparation was active and which was inert, so they could not, deliberately or inadvertently, influence the results. Such a study design, in which both the physician and the patient are unaware of the contents of a particular preparation, and both a placebo and an active drug are being used, is referred to as a "double-blind crossover." It is considered the gold standard of clinical research.

My first patient, whom I'll call George, was a frail seventy-four-year-old man with arthritis of the hips who needed a cane to get about. He complained of tightness and pressure in his chest when walking outdoors, especially in cold weather, going uphill, and after eating. A nitroglycerin tablet under the tongue relieved these symptoms in less than a minute, and he was using four or five of them every day. This is all typical of angina pectoris. Although his electrocardiogram (ECG) was normal when he was resting, it became abnormal after a stress test such as walking on a treadmill or pedaling a bicycle. These changes after exercise reflect the inability of narrowed coronary arteries to provide sufficient blood flow to the heart muscle.

At the outset of the study, I told George how enthusiastic I was about the new medication I would be giving him, and that I expected it would help him a great deal. I then handed him his first two-week supply of preparation "A," which he was to take three times a day. (I wonder whether doctors testing bowel function start with "Preparation H.") I assured him that we did not expect any serious side effects, but I asked him to report any that he might develop. I had no idea whether this first batch was active or the placebo. George left the clinic hopeful and happy.

At his next visit, fourteen days later, George was euphoric! How was his angina? What angina? He announced that he could now walk briskly without any chest discomfort whatsoever. He no longer even needed his cane! Were there any side effects? Yes, he was slightly nauseated, but that was a small price to pay for the relief he was getting. An emotional, demonstrative individual, George embraced me, kissed me, and thanked me for the "miracle."

At this point, it was obvious to me that "A" was not the placebo! Not only was it working; it was even causing some side effects, albeit minor ones. Of course, I wasn't supposed to make this observation, especially so early in the trials, since this was, after all, a double-blind study. But how could I help it, given this man's extraordinary response? I couldn't wait to see "A's" dramatic effects on the other angina patients receiving it. As the study progressed, I was surprised that some of them either did not respond at all or improved far less dramatically than George.

The study design called for objective evaluation of the drug by means of an electrocardiogram and a stress test. Remember that George's ECG had always been abnormal after the stress test. I was sure that, given the complete relief from pain afforded by this new medication, his latest ECG would show at least some improvement. But, again to my surprise, it was as abnormal as it had always been. I chalked that up to the lag we sometimes observe between the time a drug begins to work and the appearance of objective evidence. I was confident that in time our conquest of

George's angina would be reflected in an improved stress electrocardiogram.

In the second two-week phase of the study, my "miracle" patient was given tablet "B." Remember, he had no idea that this was a different pill. In my mind, the matter was settled. "B" had to be the placebo. But interestingly enough, George's symptoms did not return with "B." He remained impressively free of angina, though his stress test was still as abnormal as ever. I interpreted the continued improvement of his symptoms as a carryover effect of "A."

And so it went, switching from "A" to "B" after each two-week period—a continued improvement of symptoms but no change in the abnormal stress test.

After the study was completed, all the doctors who had participated met to evaluate the results. Just for the fun of it, each of us ventured an opinion as to which preparation we thought was the active one. There was no unanimity. Some were certain it was "A"; others were equally adamant that it was "B." Of course, only I knew for sure! We then analyzed the patients' scorecards, tallying the number of episodes of chest pain and how many nitroglycerin tablets they had taken for relief of their angina, both while on the placebo and when taking the active agent.

The moment of truth was at hand. The drug company's representative unlocked the code. My colleagues sat on the edge of their chairs waiting for the answer. I grinned like a Cheshire cat because for me the announcement would be an anticlimax. My patient had spilled the beans weeks ago. So you can imagine my shock, my disbelief, my chagrin, my disappointment, when the representative announced that "B," not "A," was the active preparation! It wasn't because my ego was deflated. I'd been wrong before. It's just that I had hoped that this new drug would turn out to be a cure for millions of people with angina. I refused to accept the verdict and asked for the "A" tablets to be analyzed by an independent laboratory. I was convinced there had been a labeling error. One week later, I received the results. "A" was indeed the placebo! George, trusting soul that he was, and I had both been led down the garden path for two solid months by our wishful expectations—he for relief of his symptoms, and I for a medical breakthrough!

Here's what else we found in this study. Symptoms of angina improved to some extent in twenty-four of the fifty patients in the study with both the placebo *and* the active pill! Such individuals are called "placebo-responders"; they feel better no matter what "medication" they are given, as long as they are convinced beforehand that it will help. Because the active drug and the blank yielded the same "improvement" under blind conditions, the agent being tested was deemed not to be effective. This conclusion was also borne out in several identical trials at other hospitals.

Are you wondering what I told George about our findings? What would you have done? Would you have continued to prescribe the placebo? I did not. I was honest with him, even though he was as incredulous and disappointed as I was with the results. But I felt it was dangerous for him to continue taking the placebo because, believing this drug to be highly effective, he might begin to wonder why he needed any other medications and be tempted to stop them, which could be very dangerous. Also, angina is nature's warning that the heart is being stressed beyond the ability of the coronary arteries to nourish it adequately. Patients who experience such chest pain almost always stop what they're doing and take a "nitro" under the tongue to ease their symptoms. This little pill dilates the coronary arteries and restores adequate blood flow to the heart muscle. The pain then goes away. George wasn't feeling any pain, because the placebo was interfering with his ability to *perceive* it. However, his heart muscle was nevertheless being deprived of the oxygen it vitally needed, as evidenced by his continued abnormal ECG response to stress-testing. Without a warning signal, he might continue to exert himself and put his life in jeopardy.

My reason for describing this dramatic response to an inert preparation is to make you aware of the placebo phenomenon. *Any health measure or intervention dispensed to a randomly selected group of individuals who are assured that it will "work" may result in improvement as often as half the time.* The response to a "dummy" pill often mimics that induced by pharmacologically active substances. For example, a placebo's effect can peak and wane, and it is almost as likely as an active substance to cause side effects. So whenever you hear testimonials ("Thanks to Preparation A, I feel like a kid again!") and anecdotal evidence ("One of my patients reported feeling better after trying Preparation A") of a sensational cure or response to any treatment, regardless of whether it's "conventional" or "alternative," always remember George and his placebo pill. Enthusiasm is no substitute for proof! Always ask whether any treatment you're considering has been properly evaluated, no matter how dramatic the testimonials.

Double-blind studies such as the one in which I participated are the best way, in most instances, to evaluate the safety and effectiveness of any new treatment in a reliable and scientific manner. But in the real world of people, suffering, and emotions, there are some conditions and treatments that simply cannot be studied in this way. It's easy enough to look at numbers when testing a drug to lower blood pressure or control high blood sugar, but how does one measure the impact of spiritual healing or meditation on someone's attitude and equanimity? Unless we bear this distinction in mind, we place an unfair and impossible burden of proof on those forms of alternative medicine that deal with such intangibles. Nor should we dismiss any kind of intervention simply because it doesn't prolong life. *Quality* of life is at least as important.

No one has yet been fully able to explain the placebo response. It's probably a combination of suggestibility, expectancy, and conditioning (previous experience with illness has primed most of us to expect that when a doctor does something—anything—it must be for our good). It may also be due to the release of natural opioids (morphine-like painkillers) from areas of the brain that are activated by certain procedures and thought processes. Several runners have died from heart attacks because they either ignored or didn't experience the warning signal of angina, presumably because of the action of these natural opioids. That may well explain George's response to preparation "A"—and the reason I stopped him from taking it. There must be other explanations too, not the least of which is the impact of the patient-therapist relationship.

Responses to a placebo are sometimes even more dramatic than what I observed in my study. For example, women who believe (because they have been so convinced, or simply because they want to) that they are pregnant may develop a bloated, pregnant-looking abdomen. They may even experience labor-like contractions! (This phenomenon, called "pseudocyesis," is caused by a poorly understood hormonal mechanism, and it occurs in other mammals too, usually after an infertile copulation.)

Placebos can relieve virtually every *subjective* symptom you can think of—including pain, nausea, hunger, fatigue, dizziness, anxiety, and depression. You name it, a placebo can fix it, at least temporarily. However, I have never known a placebo to shrink a cancerous lump, reduce a fever, lessen swelling in the legs, or eliminate fluid from the lungs of someone with heart failure. Nor, in my own experience, has it ever cured any physical, organic, "real" disease.

I used to think that I could predict who among my patients would respond to a placebo and who wouldn't. I expected that dependent personalities, people who are awed by authority figures (of which doctors are, or used to be, classic examples), who are afraid of not living up to what is expected of them, would enthusiastically respond to any treatment just in order to comply! By contrast, it seemed more likely that cynical individuals would not. But it hasn't worked out that way. Some of my most skeptical patients have reacted positively to placebos in one situation, and not in another. The truth is we are all, to some extent, suggestible. Whether or not we take the "bait" in any given trial depends very much on who is offering the cure, and on how urgently we need help.

We dispense placebos at my hospital, a university medical center. Should we be doing so? Is it right to tell patients they're being given (and, incidentally, paying for) an active drug, while providing them with "nothing"? Or is it sneaky, elitist, and dishonest? I'm not sure. I have seen placebos work in people suffering from symptoms that appear to have no physical basis or explanation. Under these circumstances, when the diagnosis is unclear, it may be safer to prescribe a placebo than a powerful drug with potential side effects. But a placebo should never be a substitute for a proven treatment that can cure an underlying problem. Now, what's the difference between a "quack" and an M.D. who prescribes blanks? Just this: The doctor uses placebos out of desperation; the quack, as you will read in chapter 3, does it to make money.

Once you are aware of the placebo effect, you can better appreciate how difficult it is to decide whether a given treatment really works. The power of the mind, and of suggestibility, is so great that many of us improve no matter what we're given. And that's fine as long as we, and our doctors, don't kid ourselves that we are really influencing the course of a disease, be it heart trouble, diabetes, AIDS, or cancer. I'm all for getting my patients to feel better, but not at the expense of really stopping a disease in its tracks. That's something placebos cannot do. It's vital to differentiate those alternative medicine approaches that function as placebos and those that are truly effective.

❖ 3 ❖

HOW TO SPOT A QUACK
There's a Sucker Born Every Minute

Double, double toil and trouble,
Fire burn and cauldron bubble.
Eye of newt, and toe of frog,
Wool of bat, and tongue of dog.

—from *Macbeth,* by William Shakespeare

Webster's dictionary defines "quack" as "a harsh, throaty cry of a duck or any similar sound." That's not the quack I have in mind in this chapter. The other definition, somewhat more to the point, is "a fraudulent pretender to medical skill, a person who pretends, professionally or publicly, to skill, knowledge or qualifications he or she does not possess; a charlatan." That's pretty accurate as far as it goes, but doesn't tell the whole picture. There are knowledgeable, qualified, and competent persons who deliberately peddle quackery because they have neither integrity nor conscience. I prefer to define a quack as someone who, for personal or financial gain, regardless of qualifications, sells, prescribes, or performs treatments that he or she *knows* to be ineffective, dangerous, or both.

It's sometimes hard to tell a legitimate though unorthodox alternative medical approach from a fraudulent "get well quick" scheme. You can't always depend on "credentials," either. Although you're much more likely to be deliberately duped by an "expert" hiding behind the anonymity of a P.O. box number than by a licensed doctor, a medical degree is no guarantee that a practitioner's recommendations are effective, safe, or offered in good faith. There are, alas, too many "reputable" physicians who have no qualms about ripping off desperate patients with expensive treatments they know to be worthless—just to make a buck. And although you should be especially wary of any anonymous sales pitch that comes to you in a gaudy, unsolicited brochure or tabloid publication, several flamboyant "health" letters filled with nonsense are peddled by licensed physicians.

I received such a newsletter a few months ago from a doctor who proudly announced that he had broken with the "establishment"—the "medical racketeers"—who are engaged in a conspiracy of silence to withhold from the American people all the wonderful things that can ensure a long and healthy life. His new mission in life was to make this advice available to anyone who would send him a mere $79.90 for a two-year subscription to his newsletter (an incredible saving of $58!). In exchange, he would let his readers in on all kinds of "amazing" medical secrets that "your doctor won't tell you." Here is one example of such a "confidential" report: "Three out of four heart patients who took yohimbine (a drug derived from the bark of the yohimbe tree in South America) had an immediate return of sexual potency after receiving heart transplants by Dr. Christiaan Barnard." I'd have thought that a man who had just been given a heart transplant, especially in those early days, would have more pressing concerns on his mind then sexual intercourse, at least for a little while. I was also surprised that any doctor would want to document transplant patients' sexual vigor at this time of their lives. And a small sample of four patients isn't statistically anything to write home about anyway. In my own practice, I have found that yohimbine "works" at best 25 percent of the time and often causes unpleasant side effects. I no longer prescribe it.

Later, in another issue of this newsletter, I was surprised to read that "common household items may be filling your body with aluminum—a *leading cause* of Alzheimer's disease." In fact, the jury is still out on that one—way out. Although it's a good idea to avoid excessive intake of aluminum, just in case, there's no basis for calling it a "leading cause" of Alzheimer's.

Perhaps the most dangerous and, in my view, most unforgivable advice proffered in this newsletter by "America's number one health advocate" was to reject coronary artery bypass surgery, which he calls useless and hazardous. Instead, he suggests a wide variety of "natural" remedies, some of which he sells through the mail. As a cardiologist, I have seen hundreds of patients whose lives have been prolonged and their quality improved by coronary bypass. For this doctor to make a blanket condemnation that will be read—and perhaps believed—by thousands to whom he has not spoken, whom he has not examined, and whose electrocardiograms, stress tests, and angiograms he has not seen—advising them to reject what may be a lifesaving procedure—is reprehensible. While this (and other) kinds of surgery are in some cases done unnecessarily, that is not a shortcoming of the procedure itself; it is a shortcoming of the doctor who has recommended it. When someone with angina pectoris (chest pain on exertion due to narrowed or obstructed coronary arteries in the heart) is not responding to medical management—diet, weight loss, regular exercise, other lifestyle changes, and medication—and the diagnosis is confirmed by an angiogram, bypass surgery, or opening the vessel with balloon angioplasty, may be essential. That newsletter's irresponsible

proselytizing from afar is the hallmark of the quack, no matter how many degrees he or she has.

There are, of course, several excellent medical newslet-
ters, such as those put out by Tufts, Berkeley, Harvard,
Johns Hopkins, and other centers of learning. Although
there are exceptions, a newsletter distributed by such an
institution is more likely to be credible than one signed by
an individual who uses it to promote a mail-order business.

You can also receive dangerous or inaccurate advice from
an otherwise reputable source who genuinely believes in
some way-out, personal pet theory. Such a practitioner is
sincere but mistaken, and his or her motive is rarely mone-
tary gain. Here are some examples.

A few years ago, a Harvard professor of the highest integrity and the best credentials began to treat angina pectoris
with radioactive iodine. His rationale was that this would
destroy the patient's thyroid gland, thus lowering the metabolism of the body and causing the heart to beat more slowly;
this would decrease the heart's workload, and eventually
improve symptoms. He was, in effect, creating one disorder
to treat another. It may sound logical on paper, but knocking
out the thyroid gland added insult to injury and actually
made all the patients who "bought" the theory much sicker.

Another, equally prestigious doctor, this one a surgeon at
a world-famous hospital in New York City, convinced some
of his colleagues that directing high-dose radiation to the
chest wall would alleviate angina by irritating the underlying heart so that it would form new blood vessels. His results
were equally disastrous.

A famous breast surgeon, William Halsted, originated an
operation that bore his name, in which an entire cancerous
breast, the underlying muscles of the chest wall, and all the
glands on the affected side were removed. This operation
was the standard procedure for treating breast cancer for

more than half a century and was abandoned only fairly recently. It unnecessarily mutilated countless women over the years, and was, in the words of my teacher and friend Dr. Ray Lawson, of McGill University, "the greatest standardized surgical error of the twentieth century."

None of these "innovators" was a quack or a fraud. However, they were all plain wrong—grievously and dangerously wrong—and their theories were ultimately abandoned. But in the interim, thousands of people suffered.

Of course, many ideas from noted scientists do pan out (consider Alexander Fleming's observation of the effect of mold on bacteria, which ushered in the era of antibiotics). And equally important contributions have been made by persons without formal scientific training. As mentioned earlier, Nathan Pritikin is a case in point. When he suggested that a low-fat, high-fiber diet, combined with regular exercise, could prevent or delay heart disease, he was scoffed at by the medical profession—simply because he wasn't a doctor. Years later, his theory became, and remains to this day, the official policy of the American Heart Association. (But oh how I wish they would also recommend fiber!)

Anyone suffering from symptoms that are difficult or even impossible to overcome by scientifically tested therapies is fair game for the quack who enters the marketplace offering a "treatment" backed up by testimonials and anecdotes, but no proof or data.

So how can you spot a quack? You should suspect quackery in the following situations.

A product promises to cure a variety of ailments quickly

Instant fixes are rare in medicine. Yes, the right antibiotic can eradicate an infection; insulin will lower very high blood sugar in diabetics; various analgesics can relieve pain promptly; acute appendicitis is curable by surgery. But these are not the problems that quacks target. They are more likely to promise to "electrify your sex life," or get you to "burn 200 calories without exercise," or "cure your fatigue"—all in no time at all. Other classic copy reads: "Say good-bye to arthritis. There is new proof that our product not only helps eliminate arthritis symptoms, but actually reverses the disease." "We have a sure cure for a weakened heart with two new over-the-counter remedies." "Let us cure your ulcer drug-free." (There are many ways to treat an ulcer, but the only way to cure it is with a combination of antibiotics that eliminate *Helicobacter pylori,* the bacterium that usually causes it.)

Testimonials and "case histories" are used to bolster claims for a particular treatment, potion, herb, or device that has allegedly alleviated or cured conditions considered incurable

Beware of "unsolicited" letters that say "I have arthritis. After taking your preparation, I'm playing golf every day. My knees are working again!" "Thanks to you, I'm beating the odds!" "I'm getting younger and better." Even when sincere, such results have other possible explanations. Remember, the severity of many disorders and diseases waxes and wanes; this is part of their "natural history." Or the improvement described may be due to the power of suggestion or the placebo effect (see chapter 2). Finally, the terrible disease that is alleged to have been cured may have been wrongly diagnosed in the first place; it may never really have existed. The best way to document the response to any given therapy is to give it to enough people and measure its effect objectively. That's something a quack never does.

A product promises overnight weight loss

The pitch here is usually the promise of rapid and sustained weight loss by means of a particular diet or supplement. No such diet exists, whether conceived in Beverly Hills or Scarsdale. Yet intelligent patients have asked me, quite seriously, whether "butter, sour cream, and salad oils melt fat," and result in "no-hunger weight loss," as claimed. These assertions are quoted verbatim from a widely distributed monthly publication in which the author states that his methods have helped "hundreds of thousands" of patients reverse and prevent illness, not to mention drop those unwanted pounds!

A product promises to grow more hair quickly

There's only one sure way to have a full head of hair—quickly—and that's to buy a wig! A weave or hair transplant takes a little longer. Over the very long term, the only preparation that *may* prevent baldness due to further hair loss is minoxidil (Rogaine)—and that's it. Any other claim, such as the one about the "three vitamins that help prevent baldness," or a lotion that promises to unclog hair follicles, is at best an exaggeration.

A treatment promises to help you look years younger

There are only three ways to prevent skin from aging or delay its aging. The first is to die young, the second is to stay out of the sun, and the third is to get a face-lift. If you're really determined to turn back the clock, the only way to do it is to reset its hands! Mind you, newer cosmetic creams and ointments can reduce wrinkling and improve the texture of your skin. But the quacks aren't pushing premium department store products! Their vitamin and nutritional supplements cost much more. Their latest focus is on antioxidants, of which you can get all you need from five to seven servings of fruit and vegetables a day. But they prefer you to fork over your money for their "special" pills, which are not nearly as good for you as the natural sources.

A product promises to increase your sexual powers and libido

This one nets a lot of fish. After all, who doesn't want to enjoy sexual peaks and desire after sixty as often (and as vigorously) as at age twenty? No problem! They've got the herb for you, whether it's straight ginseng, Baj Jee Tian tea, Strong Man Bao, Ching Chun Bao, their own brand of megavitamins and minerals, or yohimbine—all of which help you enjoy breathtaking sex! Take my advice. If you lack the desire or ability to function sexually, see a good urologist or gynecologist. He or she will check the level of your sex hormones with a simple blood test. If they're low, supplemental therapy can help; if you are diabetic, getting your blood sugar under control will sometimes improve matters; if the arteries to the male sex organs are diseased and obstructed, revascularizing them may help; if you have a psychological hang-up about sex, a good therapist can make a difference. But Strong Man Bao? Baloney!

A product or treatment boasts a "special" or secret formula for whatever purpose

It may be acceptable business practice for Coca-Cola to guard its secret formula, but soft drinks are not medications. The constituents of every product that claims to have health benefits should be disclosed on its label. When the research of a drug company bears fruit, and a worthwhile medication is discovered, it's patented, and its contents and mechanisms of action are published for the world to see. That's the way it should be. Stay away from any "health" preparation whose ingredients are not listed—no ifs, ands, or buts. Such potions usually turn out to be little more than colored water!

Ads for the potions or treatment claim to "cleanse" the body of "poisons" and "toxins" or "strengthen your immune system"

There's no such cleanser or strengthener, except for good nutrition.

A sales promotion is accompanied by a condemnation of the medical "establishment"

This is almost always the hallmark of the quack. Here is one example I came across in a "health" periodical. "Remarkable cures CENSORED by knife-happy surgeons and greedy drug companies." Or, "Medical fat cats want to CENSOR dozens of medically proven cures!" We're never told who proved them or who censored them. Even if there were some mechanism for doing so, no doctor or pharmaceutical company has the power to censor anything.

Claims are made of "persecution" by the FDA or the medical establishment

Watch out for statements like "They tried to buy me off" (without the slightest hint of who wanted to do the buying, why, or for how much). None of these attempts is ever documented. Can't you just visualize the FDA commissioner trying to buy someone's silence? Or a drug company paying off an investigator *not* to produce an effective medication? That's the kind of poppycock the quack uses to gain sympathy—the old technique of trying to win support by attacking "them."

A computerized health questionnaire scores your "nutritional deficiencies" for a hefty price

Your own doctor can best assess your nutritional state with a thorough medical history, a careful physical exam, and the appropriate tests. No computer printout interpreted by a stranger can determine your deficiency in a host of exotic chemicals. Such an "analysis" is expensive and usually worthless.

I could go on and on, listing examples of rip-offs in the making and how to spot them. But you probably get the picture.

❖ ❖ ❖   The bottom line? Look very carefully into every treatment suggested to you, regardless of its source, especially if there's any risk involved; determine how commonly it's used; ask how long it's been around; find out in what percentage of cases it has been documented to be successful; be aware of its potential side effects; and ask whether there are better or proven treatments to accomplish the same end. Finally, check to see whether it is approved by the American Medical Association (AMA), the organization that for many years has alerted Americans to fraudulent treatments, and continues to do so.

In the following chapters, we'll look at some of the more popular alternative medicine approaches, and see which ones are worth trying.

❖ 4 ❖

ACUPUNCTURE
The Needling of America

Chinese health providers have been using acupuncture for at least 5,000 years, but when I was a medical student in the 1950s, the subject was never even mentioned. My teachers considered acupuncture no more relevant to a doctor's education than a fortune cookie. Yet fifty years earlier, Sir William Osler, one of the great physicians of his time, wrote in the first edition of his classic textbook of medicine: "For lumbago, acupuncture is, in acute cases, the most efficient treatment." (He referred to acupuncture needles as "hatpins.")

It wasn't until President Nixon reestablished diplomatic relations with China, and James Reston of *The New York Times* described, in 1971, how acupuncture had eased his pain after an emergency appendectomy in China, that American doctors began to have any interest in this procedure. However, even after scrutiny that has now lasted more than twenty-five years, there is still no consensus concerning its usefulness. While some physicians are convinced that it is a panacea, others insist that it is a sham; and I suspect that most aren't sure one way or another. In their book *A Consumer's Guide to Alternative Medicine* (Prometheus Books, 1992), Kurt Butler and Dr. Stephen Barrett take an extremely negative position on acupuncture. (Barrett is a retired psychiatrist who has devoted himself to exposing medical fraud and heads a powerful antiquack organization in this country.) In their view, it is a colossal hoax, a "con" job perpetrated on the American public by Mao Zedong! They accuse him of deliberately orchestrating phony acupuncture demonstrations in order to divert attention from the shortage of doctors and the poor medical care in China. By conferring his blessing on acupuncture and designating anyone who practiced it a "doctor," Chairman Mao eliminated the shortage of doctors in China with a single stroke of the pen. According to Butler and Barrett, anyone (Reston included?) who "responds" to acupuncture must have been hypnotized, drugged, or otherwise "psyched out." I cannot reconcile this negative view of acupuncture with the experiences of countless American and other Western physicians who have seen acupuncture performed firsthand and who believe that it does work.

In my opinion, acupuncture is effective in certain circumstances. For example, it is used as an anesthetic for surgical procedures in veterinary medicine. Animals cannot be hypnotized, "psyched out," or "conned." In 1978, I was a member of a medical team that went to China to explore the possibility of scientific exchange between our two countries. We visited several Chinese health care facilities, including a university hospital in Shanghai, where I witnessed an open-heart operation—the repair of a mitral valve. The patient, a woman of about twenty-eight, was wheeled into the operating room, awake, alert, and smiling. She was "prepped" in the usual way; her chest was cleansed with an antiseptic solution. Scalpel poised, the surgeon was about to begin the procedure, when I asked in horror, "Wait a minute! What about anesthesia? Are you going to open her chest while she's awake?" "Oh, but she is already being anesthetized," he answered, pointing to the needles in the patient's left earlobe and the small electrical generator to which they were connected. "By acupuncture."

Never having witnessed acupuncture before, I was a bit apprehensive, to say the least, as the surgeon began to cut through the patient's breastbone with an electric buzz saw! After her chest was split in two, it was spread apart with a large clamp to expose the heart. The repair of the diseased valve took about thirty minutes, after which the breastbone was sewn together with steel sutures (stitches), the skin was closed, and the patient was wheeled out of the operating room—still awake!

I suspect that we were invited to that particular hospital not for a demonstration of its surgeons' skill, but to be shown that acupuncture works. Well, they certainly convinced me! What an experience! I'm a cardiologist, and I have attended scores of such heart operations, but I had never seen anything like this. (I wish Dr. Barrett had been there with me!) I would never have believed that anyone could remain wide awake, let alone smile, while her chest was being sawed open! The five other American doctors who were there with me—and my wife—were equally flabbergasted. I took a color photograph of that memorable scene: the open chest, the smiling patient, and the surgeon's hands holding her heart. I show it to anyone who scoffs at acupuncture.

Was I duped by Chairman Mao? Had this woman been given some mysterious drug that left her fully awake and alert, yet prevented the terrible pain associated with open-heart surgery? Such a medication would be even more impressive than acupuncture itself! The fact is, no such drug exists. Morphine, the strongest narcotic, can deaden most pain, but not the kind that opening the chest wall and tearing it apart would cause!

Might this patient's indifference to the pain have been explained by hypnosis? Had someone "put her under" before we came into the room? That's the explanation Victor Herbert—a doctor, distinguished researcher, author, professor of medicine, and relentless critic of quackery—would offer. According to him, "quackupuncture," as he calls it, is simply a state of heightened suggestibility, and anyone who can be easily hypnotized will also respond to acupuncture. Frankly, I've never seen hypnosis, however profound, raise anyone's threshold of pain to such a level.

To explain how acupuncture works, the ancients theorized that a life force called *ch'i* (pronounced "chee") dominates every living organism. Opposing forces within the body, designated *yin* and *yang,* must be in balance or harmony before *ch'i* can get our vital functions (spiritual, mental, physical, and emotional) to work normally. (Interestingly, the ancient Hebrews referred to this life spirit as *chai,* and modern Jews wear its symbol, shaped like an inverted "U" with a little beak on it, around the neck. They do not, however, attribute any therapeutic properties to it.)

Ch'i is said to flow along fourteen invisible, interconnected main channels ("meridians") on each side of the body, crisscrossing the arms, legs, trunk, and head, and coursing deep within the tissues. These meridians surface at various locations on the body, called "acupuncture points" ("acupoints"). At least 360 such points have been identified, and some modern acupuncturists claim that there are thousands. Each meridian "services" one or more specific organs such as the kidney, liver, gallbladder, colon, or heart, which can be influenced by stimulating the appropriate acupoints. Dietary changes, emotional stress, sexual malfunction, physical injury, unusually hard work, cancer, infection, or any of the "six pernicious influences"—wind, cold, fire, dampness, dryness, and summer heat—can interfere with or reflect an altered flow pattern of *ch'i*. The resulting imbalance between *yin* and *yang,* and the five elements of the universe—wood, fire, earth, water, and metal—cause lactic acid and carbon monoxide to accumulate in the muscles. This makes them stiff and creates abnormal pressure on the circulatory system, lymph glands, nerves, skeletal system, and other body tissues. Stimulating the appropriate acupoints dissipates the accumulated lactic acid and restores the *yin-yang* balance and the flow of *ch'i*.

Western scientists have a different explanation for acupuncture's effect. They believe that stimulating an acupuncture point causes the release of opiates, called "endorphins," within the brain. These natural substances reduce one's perception of pain as effectively as any combination of narcotics, and without the side effects of narcotics. This theory is supported by the fact that when experimental animals are given naloxone, a chemical that blocks endorphins, they do not respond to acupuncture. Dr. Herbert accepts the existence of endorphins, but he believes that any painful stimulus (such as pinching an animal's bottom, which he says he has done) will also release these endorphins, with no need for acupuncture.

There is no convincing *objective* evidence of the physical existence of meridians. However, when looked at under the microscope, acupuncture points reveal a greater concentration of nerve endings than do other skin locations. What's more, these points generate measurably more electromagnetic energy. The Chinese literature is replete with descriptions of meridians in animals and—yes—in plants, too! A paper published in 1944 in the *American Journal of Chinese Medicine* describes how acupuncture needles inserted in the stem of soybean plants and left there for two days increased the temperature in certain portions of the leaf.

Before they stick you with their needles, acupuncturists first examine your pulse. (Chances are they will also take a close look at your tongue, which they consider to be a key source of diagnostic information.) But this is no ordinary pulse-taking! Most of us are accustomed to having our pulse taken for a few seconds just to see whether it's regular, or to count it. But for the acupuncturist, a "reading" usually lasts at least several minutes, and sometimes as long as two hours. The acupuncturist places three fingers, first on one of the subject's wrists, then the other, feeling for nine pulses on each side—three deep, three intermediate, and three superficial. Each of the eighteen pulses may have as many as twenty-seven different characteristics, described in such exotic terms as "sharp as a hook," "taut as a music string," or "soft and fluttering like floating feathers blown by the wind." Several factors influence the pulse—the time of day it's taken, whether you're male or female (additionally, in women, the phase of the menstrual cycle is important), the atmospheric pressure, the temperature, the humidity, the season, and the local climate. The information thus obtained indicates the status of *ch'i* and accounts for the patient's symptoms—and their source.

Once the acupuncturist has a diagnosis, you're ready to be "needled." Acupuncture needles are almost always straight and as thin as a hair ($\frac{1}{17,000}$ to $\frac{1}{18,000}$ of an inch in diameter), and they vary in length from a fraction of an inch to several inches. Most needles are made of stainless steel or copper, but they also come in gold, silver, bamboo, and wood. (The acupuncture "staple" is round, made of metal, with a tiny needle at its end. It is attached to the ear, and left there for as long as two weeks. Staples are used mostly to control appetite, to break a bad habit, or to end an addiction such as cigarette smoking or drug abuse). Whatever their composition, make sure that the needles used on you are disposable. That's the best way to prevent the transmission of hepatitis, HIV (the virus that causes AIDS), and bacterial infections.

Depending on your condition, the acupuncturist will generally place up to twelve needles into your body about one quarter of an inch deep (the depth may vary between a tenth of an inch to seven inches) and either gently twirl or twist them by hand for fifteen to twenty minutes. The needles may also be activated by a weak electrical current or heated by burning an herb (mugwort), a technique called "moxibustion." Modern acupuncturists even stimulate the acupuncture points with sound waves and light rays of a specific wavelength. And there's no telling where the needles will be inserted—in your temple, on the bridge of your nose, the rim of your ear, or in your legs. For example, to relieve your back pain, you might have needles placed in your leg, hand, or ear. To treat circulatory problems in the head, the acupuncturist might put needles in your small toe!

You're not likely to be "acupunctured" during an acute heart attack, or if you have a bleeding problem; nor will the needle be inserted in the abdomen if you're pregnant, or into cancerous tissue, for fear of spreading it.

Acupuncture doesn't hurt; it feels very much like a mosquito bite, but it can sometimes leave you with a slight ache at the acupuncture points. Many patients describe a tingling or buzzing sensation and feel a sense of heaviness in the area, especially when the acupuncture is being done "correctly."

The number of sessions depends on the condition being treated. I have patients who've responded to an attack of acute back pain in just two sittings; others with a chronic problem see their acupuncturist at regular intervals, as they would a physiotherapist.

Instead of needling, some acupuncturists apply pressure to the designated points with their fingers and hands; some even use their knees, elbows, and feet! The Japanese have employed such "acupressure" methods for over 5,000 years. They call it *shiatsu,* and it's officially authorized in Japan by the Ministry of Health and Welfare.

There are laws or regulations governing the use of acupuncture in our fifty states. The FDA, which has recently approved the use of acupuncture as a "medical device," estimates that between 9 million and 12 million Americans are "acupunctured" each year—for a multitude of problems ranging from back pain to bladder infections. There are about 3,000 physicians nationwide who practice it (up from only 500 ten years ago); twenty-one states restrict that right to licensed doctors; the other twenty-nine and Washington, D.C., permit nonphysicians who complete a training course and pass a certifying exam to set up a "needle" shop.

Although requirements for acupuncture licensure vary, they are generally demanding. For example, in New York State, formal training consists of a three-year course (medical school is four years) at a school or college of acupuncture. The comprehensive curriculum must provide at least 1,350 hours of entry-level acupuncture education, a minimum of 800 hours of lectures and instruction, and no less than 500 hours of clinical (hands-on) training. The student must then pass a standardized final exam. So this is no correspondence course in which you can pick up a diploma after a pleasant weekend at a local hotel.

Despite the reticence, caution, conservatism—call it what you will—of the American medical establishment, the World Health Organization (WHO) lists 104 different conditions that can legitimately be treated by acupuncture—everything from pain to the common cold. But I have the impression that in most countries, and even in China these days, it is usually used only after conventional methods have failed. Even then, it's likely to be part of a "package" of complementary medicine that includes other measures such as herbal remedies or some form of relaxation therapy.

Much of the evidence for the effectiveness of acupuncture is anecdotal and subjective, but there have been several scientifically controlled studies that permit us to draw the following conclusions.

Pain management

Specialists in pain management—neurologists, physiatrists, physical therapists, and anesthesiologists—often use acupuncture in conjunction with painkillers and other conventional methods. People who suffer from chronic back pain, bursitis, osteoarthritis (especially of the knees), other musculoskeletal problems, pain after extraction of a tooth, headache, diabetic neuropathy (when the nerves have been irritated by the disease), and cancer need fewer medications and enjoy speedier recovery when treated with acupuncture. In one carefully conducted study in California, eleven women plagued by recurring menstrual cramps were treated with acupuncture once a week. The same number of controls received the usual painkillers. After three months, ten of the women in the acupuncture group had significant relief of their symptoms and were using fewer medications to control them. The others reported no change.

Asthma

Improvement of asthma after acupuncture has been measured and documented. In one Danish study of chronic asthmatics, patients experienced a 22 percent increase in airflow and a 50 percent reduction in the need for bronchial dilator drugs within two weeks after starting acupuncture. In another controlled study, almost half the subjects had no further asthmatic attacks after treatment with acupuncture. Asthmatics receiving acupuncture in a study at Oxford University reported definite improvement in their "quality of life." However, I have also read reports in which patients experienced no such improvement, and, on occasion, even noted some aggravation of their symptoms after acupuncture.

Drug abuse

The National Institute on Drug Abuse has for years been funding research on the role of acupuncture in the management of drug abuse. Some 30,000 addicts have been treated, either voluntarily or at the direction of a court, in a model study at Lincoln Hospital in New York City for the past twenty years. More than half of those receiving acupuncture did remain "clean" for at least three months, but the long-term results are not as impressive. In a similar research project in Miami, subjects treated with acupuncture stayed drug-free longer than those given "sham" therapy (needles inserted at random, rather than at designated acupuncture sites). After twenty-four months of treatment, only 3 percent of first-time offenders were arrested again in the following year for drug possession. (The usual rate of arrests is almost 60 percent in untreated addicts.) This investigation is currently being expanded, and the results continue to be encouraging. I understand that the drug court judge in Miami was so impressed with the results of acupuncture that he decided to try it himself to help break his heavy cigarette habit of twenty-five years. After ten days of acupuncture, he stopped smoking—for good!

Alcoholism

Acupuncture may be of benefit in treating severe alcoholism, at least for a while, when nothing else works. In one study, at the end of six months, treated subjects had only half as many episodes of drinking and admissions to detoxification centers as untreated patients. The investigators of this project have been awarded another grant by the NIH to evaluate the effectiveness of acupuncture in cocaine abuse, using the same study design.

Smoking

Acupuncture has been shown to help some people quit smoking. However, nicotine addiction is very powerful, and the results of acupuncture are not impressive—but then, neither is the outcome of any other techniques, including nicotine gum, nicotine patches, behavioral modification, and hypnosis. (But if you smoke, I urge you to keep trying to quit, using any or all of the above methods.)

Stroke

Stroke is the most common cause of paralysis among adults; half of its victims are left with permanent paralysis or weakness of one or more limbs. Several studies have demonstrated that acupuncture can produce a significant and measurable improvement in the physical rehabilitation of stroke survivors. Researchers in the Department of Neurology at the Boston University School of Medicine recently reported to the NIH Office of Alternative Medicine their findings in a large number of stroke patients. Those whose CT brain scans showed that less than 50 percent of their nerve pathways were damaged were left with considerably less paralysis than persons given only conventional physiotherapy. The sooner acupuncture was administered (two or three times a week for two to three months), the more effective it was. These researchers also found acupuncture effective in the treatment of paralysis from causes other than stroke, such as multiple sclerosis, Bell's palsy, and injuries to the head and neck. The scientific quality of the work was high, the latest diagnostic techniques were used, and the studies were double-blind (see chapter 2). Here, in their own words, is what the doctors concluded:

> Acupuncture appears to be helpful in the treatment of paralysis due to central nervous system damage in the majority of cases . . . when treatments are initiated in the earlier stages of paralysis. The duration of acupuncture treatments varies according to the condition being treated; it may be only a few days in treating the comatose patient, or one month when treating Bell's palsy, or 2–3 months in treating stroke patients, or 1–2 years in treating spinal cord injury cases, or even 5 years or more in treating cerebral palsy in babies and children. There were no adverse reactions reported following the acupuncture treatment for the 2,291 patients who were treated with acupuncture, across the 26 studies included in this report.

It's not clear how or why acupuncture works in these cases. It may cause the body to release greater amounts of certain hormones that dilate the arteries in the brain, improving blood flow to damaged areas, or perhaps it creates new pathways for the injured brain tissues. The important observation is that it can help prevent paralysis, and that's what counts.

Gastrointestinal disorders

A paper published in the *American Journal of Gastroenterology*—the official organ of American intestinal specialists—analyzed all the controlled studies of acupuncture in the treatment of various gastrointestinal disorders that have been reported in the Chinese and English literature. The authors of this review concluded that "there is strong evidence to support the regulatory effect of acupuncture on several gastrointestinal functions, including motility, electrical activity, and secretion." These actions are thought to take place through the same opioid mechanisms I discussed earlier. It would seem reasonable for anyone with an irritable bowel syndrome, or any other condition causing troublesome bowel symptoms resistant to conventional treatment, to try acupuncture.

Other disorders

Acupuncture is claimed to be effective in a wide variety of other disorders such as impotence; the hot flashes associated with menopause; insomnia; and nausea and vomiting during pregnancy, after surgery, or during cancer chemotherapy. The evidence of its helpfulness in treating nausea is convincing. In two studies, each involving more than 100 patients, 90 percent of subjects undergoing chemotherapy experienced relief of nausea following acupuncture. There have been several other studies in which patients given acupuncture before operations had significantly less nausea after anesthesia.

Acupuncture is still not included in the curriculum of most medical schools in this country, but the National Institutes of Health (NIH) Clinical Center in Bethesda, Maryland, is currently evaluating it. Several major hospitals use acupuncture in their pain clinics. At least eighty private insurance companies and state Medicaid programs now reimburse for this treatment, especially for the relief of acute or chronic back pain. The cost of an acupuncture session currently ranges from $40 to $100, depending on who performs it and where it's done. Physician acupuncturists usually charge more than the others. If you want to look into the legal status of acupuncture where you live and determine who will reimburse you for it, write to the National Commission for the Certification of Acupuncturists (NCCA) at 1424 16th Street, N.W., Suite 501, Washington, D.C. 20036; or phone them at 202-232-1404. To find a doctor-acupuncturist near you, call the American Academy of Medical Acupuncture at 800-521-2262; for the name of a licensed practitioner who may or may not be a doctor, contact the American Association of Acupuncture and Oriental Medicine at 610-433-2448.

Acupuncture appears to be safe, provided the needles are sterile and disposable, and you incur little risk by trying it. It doesn't always work; but then again, what treatment— conventional or alternative—has a perfect track record? If the first round isn't successful, try another therapist. Skills in this area vary considerably. And remember, the acupuncturist needn't be Chinese.

❖ ❖ ❖   Here's the bottom line. Despite the dramatic scene I witnessed in that operating room in Shanghai, it is not an ideal anesthetic. It works in only 20 percent of cases of major surgery, and is not nearly as effective or predictable as the modern, sophisticated agents and nerve blocks developed in the West. In fact, Chinese surgeons don't use acupuncture anesthesia very often and usually give additional painkillers when they do—just to be sure. But that's not the point. The question is not how good an anesthetic acupuncture is, but whether or not it can control pain in certain situations. In my opinion, the answer to that question is "yes."

I suggest that you stay with conventional anesthesia if you're having major surgery. But if you've got a bad back or some other chronic disorder that's giving you round-the-clock pain; if you suffer from asthma or irritable bowel; if you're addicted to alcohol, tobacco, or drugs; or if chemotherapy is giving you intolerable nausea, try acupuncture from a qualified practitioner. If you've had a stroke, or suddenly develop weakness or paralysis of a limb, ask your doctor or neurologist about early acupuncture. The data here are impressive.

❖ 5 ❖

APPLIED KINESIOLOGY

Is Muscle Weakness
a Diagnostic Strength?

Applied kinesiology (AK), an offshoot of chiropractic (see chapter 12), was introduced in 1964 by George Goodheart, an American chiropractor. While the rest of his colleagues remained adamant that poor alignment of the spine was the cause of most health problems, Goodheart insisted that abnormal posture, independent of alignment, was the real villain. It was his basic premise that a common hormonal, blood, nerve, or lymphatic supply—all controlled by the same meridians described in acupuncture (see chapter 4)—connects the muscles with the internal organs, and that muscle function reflects and determines physical and emotional health. According to practitioners of AK, when a muscle goes into spasm or becomes weak, we should look for and correct some other underlying disorder. They believe that, along with hair analysis (whose accuracy is seriously questioned by the conventional medical community), AK can diagnose various allergies, deficiencies, toxic states, and food sensitivities.

Advocates of AK insist that it is a very complicated, sophisticated technique requiring extensive training and experience. But although much of the muscle testing in AK appears to be subtle and complicated, some of it strains my credulity.

For example, here is how a practitioner of AK might evaluate your sensitivity to a particular food or drug. You stand with one arm by your side and the other outstretched, palm down. With a quick movement, lasting only a second or two, the therapist pushes down on your wrist, forcing your outstretched arm down. How much resistance he or she encounters establishes your "baseline." You then chew a food or some other substance to which you may be allergic or intolerant, or you hold it in your mouth long enough for it to mix with your saliva. Now, the therapist again pushes your arm down. If you are sensitive to the substance being tested, much less power is needed to force it to your side. The food or medication being evaluated can be placed in your hand instead of your mouth. For example, you could hold a penicillin or aspirin tablet, or anything else that's suspect, in one hand while the strength of the other is tested. Replenishing the substance in which you are allegedly deficient, such as potassium or sodium, supposedly makes the arm stronger.

AK practitioners insist that their diagnostic methods are at least as accurate as skin testing, blood analyses, and the other conventional methods used to identify food and drug sensitivities and deficiencies. They claim they can usually pinpoint the problem in one session, though complicated cases may require more. They also contend they can improve the quality of your life by identifying what kind of music and colors you should favor—all this by testing your muscle strength and muscular reactions.

In *Alternative Medicine,* an exhaustive but, alas, uncritical compendium published in 1994, the Goldberg Group quotes Dr. Robert Blaich, a prominent chiropractor and kinesiologist, as saying that he is able to diagnose a wide variety of disorders of the muscles, glands, or organs by means of such muscle testing, and then restore health by using one of many techniques such as joint manipulation and mobilization, myofascial therapies (myofascia is the tissue that wraps around muscles), adjustment of the head, acupuncture, and diet. For example, the strength of the deltoid muscle in the shoulder is said to be a reliable indicator of lung function, since the shoulder and lung are close to one another and have common reflex stimulation. Thus if a patient has a weak shoulder, the kinesiologist looks very carefully at his or her lungs. When the muscle and lungs are treated, both will supposedly improve.

Are the claims made for these tests valid? In searching the published scientific literature for documentation, I did not find a single study supporting either the theory on which applied kinesiology is based or the benefits attributed to it. In a report published in the *Journal of the American Dietetic Association,* different therapists performed the same maneuver on different subjects under the same conditions, and came up with varying and unpredictable results. They concluded that AK is neither accurate nor reproducible.

However, to ensure that this negative assessment of AK and the lack of published data confirming its efficacy were not a result of its being ignored by "establishment" scientific literature, I also reviewed the complementary medical literature. I found many anecdotes of miraculous improvement and cures, but few, if any, facts—and no proof. That may be why, even though its adherents are vocal, enthusiastic, and insistent about its legitimacy, AK is not widely used. Only a minority of chiropractors employ it; most insist adamantly that correcting a "malaligned spine" is the way to go, and that pushing down an outstretched arm to make a diagnosis, and then treating the problem with myofascial therapy or acupuncture, is *not*.

Out of curiosity, I tried the arm-testing technique on several patients with food allergies—and even on myself. I was unable to find any difference in the strength of their arms or mine before and after exposure to substances that didn't sit well with us. I have never personally observed weakness of the deltoid muscle in someone with pneumonia or any other lung disease, nor would I substitute AK for antibiotic therapy in such cases.

❖ ❖ ❖ The bottom line? Applied kinesiology, although it is an offshoot of chiropractic, is used by only a minority of chiropractors. Claims for its effectiveness in the diagnosis and treatment of disorders, other than those directly affecting the muscle themselves, are not substantiated by a review of all the available evidence. If you have a health problem, AK is not the way to solve it.

Note

Don't confuse kinesiology with *applied kinesiology*. The former is a proven technique of muscle testing, training, coordination, and rehabilitation that is widely and effectively used by athletes and dancers, and in the treatment of sports injuries. Several hospitals and physiotherapy institutes have departments of kinesiology, but they do not perform applied kinesiology—nor do they claim to be able to cure anything but the muscle problem.

❖ 6 ❖

AROMATHERAPY

Do Scents Make Sense?

Scents are an integral and important part of our lives. Everyone has his or her favorite aromas—a perfume or an aftershave, a bouquet of flowers, the fresh mint and tarragon in a salad, the oil used in a relaxing massage. A particular scent often brings back memories, both pleasurable and painful. The taste of cloves reminds me of childhood visits to the dentist, who dabbed clove on a tooth he'd just drilled; the aroma of Rum and Maple pipe tobacco brings my father to mind; Arpège perfume stirs reminiscences of a teenage crush when I promised her anything but. . . . Freud believed that living in urban areas deprives us of many wonderful aromas emanating from the earth, and that this, in part, is responsible for the increase in our neuroses. (And for all those years, I thought it was my mother!)

Incense and aromatic oils have been used for millennia—not just as perfumes, but to enhance religious rituals, for embalming, or simply to mask unpleasant odors. In addition, many cultures—Egyptian, Greek, Roman, Arab, Indian, Chinese—have also employed aromatic plants for health purposes: from warding off the plague to repelling disease-carrying insects. In my family, we burn citronella candles on the terrace to fend off mosquitoes; we keep bags of lavender in the closets to deter moths. My wife rids her orchids of fungus infections by putting crushed fresh ginger on their leaves.

It wasn't until the 1920s, though, that aromatherapy became a formal discipline within health care. It happened serendipitously when René-Maurice Gattefosse, a French chemist working in the perfume industry, burned his hand very badly. The only "therapy" immediately available to him was a container of pure lavender oil into which he plunged his scorched hand. To his surprise, the pain and redness subsided very quickly, and Gattefosse claimed that the burn healed within hours without leaving a scar. The chemist attributed this salutary effect to the healing and antiseptic properties of the lavender oil. He experimented with several other oils and decided that they too had potential for healing a variety of skin disorders. Other French physicians, notably Dr. Jean Valnet, began to use aromatic oils not only for skin problems but for other medical disorders as well, such as anxiety and insomnia. Valnet, who served as an army surgeon during World War II, treated burns and other wounds with essential oils such as clove, thyme, and chamomile. He also found that certain fragrances alleviated some psychiatric problems. His landmark book, *The Practice of Aromatherapy,* has been translated into English (Healing Arts Press, Rochester, Vermont, 1980, 1990). Today, France remains the center of the fragrance industry, not only for the manufacture of its famous perfumes, but also for the production of some forty

"essential" oils. These oils are aromatic, volatile, flamma-
ble substances extracted from flowers, roots, bark, leaves,
wood resins, and lemon or orange rinds. They are sprayed
into the air and inhaled, or absorbed through the skin via
massage, in hot baths, or from hot or cold compresses.
Some essential oils are also taken internally, but this is
very risky, because several are toxic when ingested. The
most important essential oils are hydrocarbons (terpenes)
and oxygenated compounds, including alcohols, ketones,
and phenols. They are extracted in concentrated form;
but by the time you buy them—so that they can be used
safely—they have been combined with other vegetable or
"carrier" oils such as soy, evening primrose, or almond, or
have been diluted in alcohol.

Don't confuse medical aromatherapy with the multi-
billion-dollar perfume and cosmetics industries. The main
purposes of perfume and cosmetics are to have you smell
good, make you socially acceptable, and enhance your sex
appeal. Professional aromatherapists claim that, in addition
to all these pluses, their substances also improve your mood
and promote good health. For them, every oil either soothes
and relaxes or stimulates and invigorates. It does so chemically, by reacting with hormones and enzymes after it enters
the bloodstream; psychologically, because of the memories it
evokes; and physiologically, because of its effect on your
pulse, blood pressure, and so on. For example, cloves, rosemary, lavender, and mint stimulate the salivary glands; cam-
phor, calamus, and hyssop oils are good for the heart and
circulation; other aromatics act on the lymphatic, endocrine,
nervous, and urinary systems; oils such as bergamot, lavender, and juniper have antiseptic properties, and, when
applied to the skin, are said to help a variety of dermatologic
disorders. The different action of each of these oils is attributed to the response of the plants from which they were

extracted to the sun, moon, earth rain, and other factors in their environment. Arnica, for example, which allegedly helps relieve the pain of bruises and athletic injuries, comes from high in the mountains, where the sun is strong and the air clean; it is said to arouse the senses and stimulate the circulation. By contrast, olive oil, whose fruit blossoms under the hot Mediterranean sun, warms and soothes.

Although aromatherapy is still more popular in Europe, especially in France, than it is in America, its use is growing in this country. Some of my patients would rather take a few drops of peppermint to ease their indigestion than use more modern (and expensive) drugs; eucalyptus is a popular additive to a humidifier (or to a bowl of water, to be inhaled under a towel) for relief of asthmatic congestion. Here are some other favorite applications of aromatherapy.

- *Massage,* usually for relief of muscle sprain or soreness. Most preparations used for this purpose (such as clary sage, chamomile, and lavender) contain only a small amount of the active ingredient blended with a light base oil such as almond or grape-seed (up to five drops per tablespoon). Higher concentrations can irritate the skin. It's not a good idea to have your massage before going out into strong sunlight or using a sunlamp, because these oils often leave the skin more sensitive to ultraviolet radiation. The same is true of many oils and lotions applied to the skin without massage. Never put them on undiluted— except for lavender oil, which can be used undiluted in small amounts to treat a burn or an insect bite.
- If you enjoy luxuriating in a *bath* with aromatic oils, don't add more than eight drops, and do so only after the bath is full and the temperature is where you want it. Bath oils can be irritating. Avoid all of them if you have any kind of skin allergy or other skin disorder.

- To relieve *muscle aches and pains* with a compress of aromatic oil, add five drops to a bowl of the water in which you are going to dip the cloth for the compress.
- You can *freshen the air* in your environment, or add a pleasant aroma to it, with commercially available spray units. But many aromatic oils require a special burner, which should be kept out of the reach of children.

Do aromatic oils help serious disease? Are there any conditions in which they're uniquely effective? If so, how do they work?

Smell is the most acute of all our senses. When there is an odor or aroma in the air, it wafts over and activates smell receptors dangling in our upper nasal passages. These thin, hairlike receptors "wear out" and are renewed every thirty days when we're young, but less frequently as we age, and often not at all in the elderly—which is why so many older people lose their sense of smell. Once activated, these receptors send nerve impulses directly to the limbic system in the brain: the seat of memory, emotion, and sexual arousal. How we respond when exposed to a particular aroma—with love, hate, rising libido, anxiety, sadness—influences our heart rate, our blood pressure, our breathing, and possibly our immune system as well. The combination of these actions can have some impact on the course of a given disease or disorder, but there is little if any evidence that it plays an important role in the management of serious disease.

Claims

Here are some of the claims proponents of aromatherapy make about its attributes and uses.

Infections

"Essential oils have antimicrobial properties." The paper on which this claim was based was written in 1958, and referred to an effect observed in the test tube, not in humans or even animals. Most similar claims also have sparse documentation. In one volume on aromatherapy, one of its most prominent advocates, R. B. Tisserand, a French doctor, states that essential oils in the proper combination stimulate the immune system. He then recommends sandalwood oil for sore throats and laryngitis, and oils of cinnamon and eucalyptus for their antimicrobial properties in respiratory infections. I love its aroma in my aftershave, but I would hesitate to use sandalwood oil for laryngitis for fear of masking a strep throat, the best treatment for which remains penicillin or a related antibiotic. In fact, I can't think of a single infection for which I would advise aromatherapy rather than an appropriate antibiotic.

Shingles

The rash caused by shingles is said to respond dramatically to equal parts of a blend of *Ravensera aromatica* and *Calophyllium inophyllum* within seven days. I have not seen any scientific documentation of that claim. The pain of shingles can be relieved to some extent by topical application of capsaicin, a substance derived from hot peppers, but I know of no topical treatment—oil, lotion, cream, or ointment—that heals the rash. So I have no objection to your trying the aromatics, but I'd take oral acyclovir (Zovirax) as well.

Arthritis

Rubbing cloves, cinnamon, thyme, or everlast and eucalyptus into an arthritic joint is said to ease the symptoms by stimulating the adrenal glands to produce more of their cortisone-like hormones. I've never seen proof of this claim, but these oils are worth trying because they do not have the cumulative toxic effect of many antiarthritic medications. Even if they do not eliminate pain, they may reduce the amount of conventional painkillers needed to control it.

Results of Studies

Here are what some scientifically valid studies report on aromatherapy.

Sleep

In a recent report in *The Lancet,* elderly patients who required substantial doses of sleeping pills slept like babies when a lavender aroma was wafted into their bedrooms at night.

Behavior

There is considerable evidence that fragrant compounds and essential oils do affect behavior. For example, mice made hyperexcitable by large amounts of caffeine were calmed by fragrances of lavender, sandalwood, and other oils sprayed into their cages. On the other hand, they became more irritable when exposed to the aroma of orange terpenes, thymol, and certain other substances. These oils were all detected in the bloodstream of the animals one hour after exposure. Experiments are currently under way to see whether pumping pleasant scents into subways will reduce violent crime there.

Stress

An equally relevant experiment was conducted at Memorial Sloan-Kettering Hospital in New York. Patients undergoing magnetic resonance imaging (MRI) often complain of claustrophobia when they are placed in a confined space—the magnetic capsule—and their movement is severely restricted during the entire procedure, which can take an hour or so. After exposure to the aroma of vanilla, patients reported that they were 63 percent less claustrophobic. (Ah, the mysteries of science! How did they know it was exactly 63 percent, and not, say, 59?) Interestingly, there were no corresponding changes in their heart rate. So the patients' anxiety was lessened either by the intensity of the pleasant memories evoked by the vanilla aroma—a purely psychological phenomenon—or by some undefined physiological response.

In another study of 122 patients under obvious stress in an intensive care unit, patients felt much better when they were given aromatherapy with oil of lavender than when they simply rested or had a massage. Again, as in the Sloan-Kettering study, the patients showed no objective changes in their blood pressure, respiration, or heart rate. (I am so impressed by these studies that I have been thinking of spraying my own waiting room with oil of lavender. I haven't done so yet, because I worry that my office staff will become sedated.) In Japan and elsewhere, fragrances are being introduced into the workplace to increase productivity. I have not as yet seen any reports about the effectiveness of this approach.

Postpartum discomfort

In a double-blind study (see chapter 2) of 635 women who added lavender oil to their bath to relieve discomfort in the perineal area (between the vagina and the rectum) after childbirth, the women noticed a distinct improvement between the third and fifth day, when these symptoms are usually worst.

Colds

In my opinion, there's no more effective and pleasurable treatment for the common cold than a bowl of chicken soup, especially the way my mother used to make it. After all, 40 million Jewish mothers who have been touting the benefits of chicken soup over the centuries (ever since Maimonides first recommended it in the twelfth century) can't all be wrong. How does chicken soup work its magic? Is it simply the steam, or the ingredients, or its beguiling aroma? In a study published in 1978, the effect on the nasal mucosa (lining of the nostrils) of inhaling steam from hot water was compared with breathing the vapors from hot chicken soup. The soup won, hands down!

Erectile function

Men, is it all in your head if your girlfriend's perfume turns you on? Or is the effect operative lower down in the body? According to research on thirty-one male volunteers, certain aromas were shown to increase blood flow to the penis, a sine qua non for a satisfactory erection. The following combinations all significantly enhanced the circulation to this organ: licorice or lavender with pumpkin pie (is that how the Pilgrims endured the long winters?); doughnut with black licorice. The most effective cologne for this purpose was one containing lavender. Men considered to be the most sexually active responded best to lavender, cola, and oriental spice, while older males preferred vanilla. Again, no one knows how these aromas produce such miracles, whether it's a Pavlovian response (like dogs reacting to a bell), or because these scents reduce anxiety. Whatever the mechanism, these findings suggest that inhalant therapies may have a role in the treatment of impotence due to blood vessel disease or psychogenic ("all in the head") factors.

Caveats

If you're considering aromatherapy, or are already using it, there are certain caveats of which you should be aware:

- Aromatic oils vary in quality, and their production is not regulated. So make sure your source is reliable. Discuss it with the vendor. Determine whether the company has been making the product for any length of time. Buying an oil from the same manufacturer or distributor makes it more likely that you will get a standardized product. Always ask for the purest available brand.
- Do not consume aromatic oils. Some can be toxic.
- Store aromatic oils in a cool place. Some, such as jasmine and neroli, should be refrigerated. Most retain their potency for two to three years, but citrus oils "die" in a year.
- With the exception of topical lavender oil for burns or insect bites, never use concentrated, undiluted oil. Refer to a good book on aromatherapy for instructions on diluting an oil.
- If your skin is sensitive, always apply a very small amount of the diluted oil before you try the whole treatment, to make sure you're not allergic to it. Five percent of the population reacts adversely to aromatic oils.
- Keep all aromatic oils away from children.
- Always close your eyes when inhaling an aromatic oil. Its "fumes" can be irritating at close range. Don't apply any oils close to your eyes.
- Do not use mint oils at night, because they can cause insomnia.
- Avoid oils of sweet fennel and rosemary if you have epilepsy. These substances may increase the excitability of the brain and induce seizures.

- If you're pregnant, avoid oils of arnica, basil, clary sage, cypress, juniper, myrrh, sage, and thyme. Some obstetricians believe that these oils can cause the uterus to contract. A woman who is at risk of a miscarriage, or who has abnormal bleeding, should keep away from chamomile and lavender. If the doctor okays it, a pregnant woman may use dilute oils of peppermint, rose, and rosemary after the fourth month.
- People with high blood pressure should avoid oils of rosemary, sage, and thyme.

There are many basic texts on aromatherapy. I found *The Herbal Body Book* by Jeanne Rose especially interesting reading. Lotus Light (P. O. Box 1008, Wilmot, WI 53710; telephone 414-889-8501) is another good source of informational materials on the subject. The Pacific Institute of Aromatherapy in San Rafael, California, and the National Association for Holistic Aromatherapy in Boulder, Colorado, can also provide you with more information.

❖ ❖ ❖   The bottom line? I don't believe aromatherapy is a major player in the fight against disease, but certain essential oils can relieve stress, can help manage some skin disorders, and are extremely pleasant.

❖ 7 ❖

AYURVEDA

Vata, Pitta, or *Kapha,* Anyone?

Westerners in general, and Americans in particular, have long been fascinated by Eastern cultures and Eastern mysticism. "Wise men" from Asia and elsewhere have plied their stock-in-trade from coast to coast throughout most of this century. (Either there aren't any "wise women," or they just aren't being exported to this country.) Despite—or perhaps because of—our much higher standard of living, our longer life span, and all the scientific and technological advances of the West, we still look to other cultures for something that can best be described as "peace of mind." That quest should be sending a message to doctors. Perhaps it has something to do with the importance of the quality of life as well as its duration; with the need to make compassion the handmaiden of technical excellence; to listen to sick people as well as give them orders. In my opinion, Eastern medical philosophies and approaches, because they make hope and humanity an integral part of health care, have become increasingly popular, despite a perceived lack of scientific review.

Ayurvedic medicine is one of these schools. I doubt that many people had even heard of Ayurveda ten years ago, let alone understood what it is all about. Since that time, however, Deepak Chopra has written so much on different aspects of this subject that many thousands now are interested in it, practice it, or are treated by its practitioners, here and abroad.

The system of healing called Ayurveda (*ayu* means "life"; *veda* means "knowledge of") originated in India sometime around 1500 B.C., although some people say there are references to it in writings dating back to 6000 B.C. Eighty percent of the population of India currently receives medical care from Ayurvedic practitioners. The basis of Ayurveda is natural healing, the belief that human beings are an integral part of nature, governed by the same principles that determine the survival and health of all living matter— plant and animal. Its goal is to bring humans into harmony or equilibrium with their environment. This concept is common to other Eastern healing disciplines, although the language and details may differ.

According to Ayurveda, every human being is a unique combination of mind, body, senses, and soul. The concepts of mind (analogous to brain or thought), body, and senses are easy to grasp. The average Westerner, however, may have trouble defining "soul." Ayurveda considers "soul" to be a vital energy—called *prana,* analogous to the Chinese *ch'i*— that leaves the body when we die. We need not go into the more philosophical aspects of this school of learning, but the soul is thought to move from body to body. So you and I may have been around for millennia and may once have been, say, Joan of Arc or Henry VIII. When someone dies, his or her "soul" inhabits another body. You can see how comforting this belief can be, especially when one is facing a life-threatening illness or is saddened by death.

While "life" comprises mind, body, senses, and soul, each of us is born with a constitution (*pakriti*) composed of varying amounts of three *doshas,* or forces: *vata,* symbolized by air or space; *pitta,* fire; and *kapha,* represented by earth and water. Your type is your individual *tridosha,* your combination of these three *doshas*—you might be predominantly *vata,* or *pitta,* or *kapha;* or *vata-kapha, pitta-kapha,* or *pitta-vata-kapha.* (Sounds like something out of an old Danny Kaye movie, doesn't it?) These characteristics, with which you're born, determine what you should eat and how you should conduct your life.

The main objective of an Ayurvedic doctor is to characterize or define your *tridosha* and prescribe accordingly. Since no two people are identical, each prescription for life and health must be individually tailored. As a general rule, those who are of a predominantly *vata* (air) constitution are full of energy and always on the move. They are most likely to be troubled by excessive gas, a bad back, arthritis, and diseases of the nervous system. *Pitta* types (fire) are volatile, quick to anger, aggressive, and competitive. Their major complaints are more likely to involve problems with the skin or liver, inflammation of some part of the body, ulcers, and gallbladder disease. *Kaphas* (earth and water) are similar to what conventional doctors call a type B personality—slower, relatively solid, and tranquil. They are more susceptible to respiratory conditions such as bronchitis and pneumonia.

Ayurvedic practitioners are trained in diet, cooking, and meditation. They also have at their disposal a veritable storehouse of different herbs. Their nutritional recommendations differ from those of the American Heart Association or the American Cancer Society in that they are not designed to be followed by populations; rather, they vary from individual to individual, on the basis of particular personal characteristics, and on how much the *tridosha* is out of whack. So Ayurvedics devise a diet for each constitutional type. In formulating these diets, how the food tastes is more important than its composition. Ayurveda recognizes six major categories of taste: (1) sweet, (2) sour, (3) salty, (4) bitter (such as leafy green vegetables), (5) astringent (such as pomegranate or beans), and (6) pungent (such as spicy, hot foods made with peppers). Sweet, sour, and salty foods raise *kapha* and lower *vata;* sweet, bitter, and astringent foods decrease *pitta,* but sour, salty, and pungent foods increase it. Don't worry—you needn't commit these to memory, because the manipulation of the diet requires specialized information best offered by a trained practitioner of Ayurveda.

But Ayurveda involves more than just diet. It also considers where someone with a particular constitutional type should live, and even what clothes he or she should wear. If you're suffering from too much *vata,* you'll probably be advised to watch less TV; but if you're a *kapha* type, you'll be encouraged to wallow as a couch potato. Failure to recognize and guide a specific combination of *doshas* can lead to an imbalance of *vata, pitta,* or *kapha.* Illness is the result of this deviation from nature.

Most alternative medicine approaches focus to some extent on elimination and detoxification—and Ayurveda is no exception. This aspect of Ayurveda is called the *three malas:* the detoxification and elimination of sweat, urine, and feces. As you will see below, every Ayurvedic regimen includes several key steps that are considered absolutely necessary to rid your body of these "poisons." These steps can be arduous.

Most Ayurvedic centers, especially those run by the Maharishi Mahesh Yogi (he's the Indian spiritual leader who introduced TM—transcendental meditation—to this country), also emphasize meditation of some kind as part of their treatment program.

Ayurveda is, by its very nature, directed more toward prevention than to treatment of disease. It also has an obvious and simplistic appeal to anyone who is stressed out and chronically fatigued. All you need to do is change the way you eat, move to another town, switch jobs, and relax. Most of my own patients would find it difficult to follow those instructions, at least on short notice. But some of the advice is reasonable, feasible, and very much what your own conventional doctor would tell you. For example, if you're tired (assuming that your thyroid function has been evaluated and found to be normal), you should get more sleep. A warm oil massage at bedtime will help you do so. Eat lighter, more easily digestible foods; add some fun to your life; avoid too much caffeine and alcohol; and stay away from fried and greasy foods. The Ayurvedics have some other interesting tips. In addition to these reasonable suggestions, they believe that cold drinks and iced foods are bad for you. The explanation—and it is a perfectly logical one but never documented—is that when cold food or liquid reaches the stomach, it causes the blood vessels there to constrict, thus impairing the speed of the digestive process (which depends on an adequate blood supply). They think a glass of hot water two or three times a day will work wonders. My mother thought so too, and she lived to be ninety-four.

But *food* is the focus of Ayurveda, whether it's concerned with allergies, bad skin, poor digestion, faulty respiration, or impaired circulation. Although much of the advice does overlap with what you would receive from a mainstream doctor, there are myriad interesting twists and taboos. The details are beyond my expertise and the scope of this book. However, I do want you to know what you're letting yourself in for when you sign up for an Ayurveda session.

When you consult a specialist in Ayurveda, in addition to a description of your actual symptoms, you will be asked about your family dynamics, job situation, and other interpersonal relationships. However, what separates the men from the boys among the Ayurvedics, and the most important skill they boast, is taking the pulse. This is a very delicate maneuver from which they assess the state and interaction of the three *doshas* in your body. Three main pulses are identified, one for each of the three doshas, and each contains several components. The trained Ayurvedic doctor claims to be able to diagnose internal disease using the pulse alone as accurately as a conventional physician can with X rays and other sophisticated equipment.

Once the cause of your illness is determined, you're likely to be treated, not with antibiotics, chemotherapy, or surgery (although the latter is permitted when necessary), but by dietary manipulation, along with a regimen of herbal supplements: powders, potions, pills, tinctures, teas, pastes, jellies, oils, and mixtures from plants and animals. Don't bother asking your pharmacist about them—or your doctor, for that matter. It's a field unto itself.

Depending on the particular setting you choose for your treatment, you're more than likely to be given massage, often with warm sesame oil, for which I have great respect ever since my patient with the tongue cancer used it so successfully (see chapter 1). (Sesame oil is also recommended in Ayurveda as a mouthwash, and some of my patients have told me they relax with *shirodhara,* the technique of having sesame oil trickle steadily down the forehead.) Ayurvedics will identify certain points of the body, called *marmas,* using techniques not unlike those of acupuncturists, and massage them. You'll also be taught breathing exercises, a favorite method being to inhale and exhale, first out of one nostril, then out of the other, for five minutes.

Then comes one of the most important procedures in Ayurveda, which I mentioned earlier. During *panchakarma,* as it is called, you undergo a series of steps in detoxification for a period lasting from days to weeks. These steps include therapeutic vomiting to cleanse the stomach and thoracic cavity; purgation, usually with castor oil, to facilitate elimination from the small intestine; vigorous enemas, often with herbal preparations, to eliminate "toxins" (the quotation marks are mine); herbal nose drops to remove more toxins from the head and sinuses; warm oil massages; and saunas, or steam baths, to which herbs are added to produce healing vapors—again, to rid your body of toxic substances. After that, you'll be gradually introduced to a diet designed especially for you.

I was unable to find any scientific proof that Ayurveda is effective against disease—it's all anecdotal. However, the recently created Office of Alternative Medicine of the National Institutes of Health has, to its credit, appointed several representatives of Ayurveda to its committees and is supporting research on Ayurvedic principles and practices. Currently, this research includes a follow-up of two matched groups: one group is using meditation, an Ayurvedic diet, and yoga postures (yoga is an important offshoot and component of Ayurvedic medicine [see chapter 9]); the other group is being treated by conventional Western methods such as a low-fat, low-salt diet and brisk walking. In another project, an Ayurvedic herbal formula is being evaluated in the treatment of Parkinson's disease, the theory being that the alkaloids in the herbs may have an important effect on the nervous tissue affected in this disease. Researchers in California are examining the benefits of Ayurvedic breathing exercises in psychiatric disorders; and in Massachusetts, researchers are investigating the potential benefit of yoga in treating heroin addiction. These studies are in progress, and no conclusions, one way or another, have yet been made. Dr. Andrew Weil, in his book *Spontaneous Healing,* states that an Ayurvedic preparation called *triphala,* with which I have no personal experience, is one of the best bowel regulators he has ever encountered and has little if any toxicity.

Other studies conducted by Ayurvedic doctors, but not evaluated or confirmed by Western scientists, have suggested that herbs used in Ayurveda may be helpful for some forms of cancer, heart disease, acne, and diabetes. The medical establishment is just beginning to look at them, and there has been no scientific documentation of which I am aware.

In the minds of most Western-trained physicians, much of what Ayurveda teaches—the importance of avoiding stress and fatigue, living a life of moderation and happiness—is old hat, and no different from what the establishment recommends. On the other hand, Ayurveda also includes what seems to me to be nonsense and is not likely to be adopted by many Americans. As a case in point, consider the advice on how to prevent cataracts: brush your teeth (okay so far), scrape your tongue (I'm beginning to wonder), then spit into a cup of water and wash your eyes with the mixture. Other Ayurvedic advice is to treat alcoholism by eating goat excrement that's been washed with urine; to drink a mixture of milk and urine to relieve constipation; to treat yourself to an enema of urine and ground-up peacock testicles for impotence; and to take enemas of animal blood to manage hemorrhage. (In all fairness, though, none of these prescriptions is part of modern Ayurveda, at least as it's practiced in this country.) Furthermore, the majority of mainstream medical doctors do not think that the *vata, pitta, kapha* classification is valid.

In brief, in addition to recommending some things that are good and are common knowledge, Ayurveda also recommends some steps that are bizarre and possibly harmful—and it prescribes some unproved therapies which should not, in the opinion of the establishment, be used. Certainly, mainstream doctors are concerned that patients will forgo proven remedies to try unproven Ayurvedic treatments instead. Positive thinking is to be encouraged, but it does not demonstrably cure cancer or any other disease. That's the position of most modern doctors with regard to Ayurveda at this time in this country.

❖ ❖ ❖   What's the bottom line? Should you head straight for an Ayurvedic clinic for indoctrination into this ancient Indian school of medicine? The answer, in a word, is no. Should you maintain an interest in its principles and recommendations for a positive lifestyle? Definitely. For example, meditation, one of the cornerstones of Ayurveda, helps me and my patients relax, though whether it prevents or cures disease is a moot point. I personally have seen no evidence that it does, although it can sometimes lower an elevated blood pressure when done regularly. But all the dietary fiddle-faddle about *vata, pitta,* and *kapha* should be taken with a grain of salt (provided, of course, you don't have high blood pressure or heart failure). Drinking urine, or soaking anything in it, is like coffee, not my cup of tea, so to speak; neither are the detoxification routines. Moreover, since Ayurveda isn't recognized as a medical discipline in this country and is therefore not licensed, it's hard to find and evaluate a practitioner. However, many of them are osteopaths, chiropractors, naturopaths, nurses, or even M.D.s who provide other forms of health care, whose credentials you can check. As far as their competence in Ayurveda is concerned, you can contact the College of Maharishi Ayur-Veda Health Center, P. O. Box 282, Fairfield, IA 52556; telephone 515-472-5866. You might also get some firsthand reports at your local Indian restaurant or grocery store.

❖ 8 ❖

BEE VENOM THERAPY
Hi, Honey, I'm Home

Like most people, I quickly change course when approached by a bee (or wasp, or mosquito, or, for that matter, any winged creature). It's not because I'm a coward, or even allergic. It's just that I can do without the pain, swelling, and itching of a bee sting. I have armed and equipped my terrace with all manner of deterrents, from special candles to insect swatters, to protect myself and my loved ones; when my family and I are outdoors, we apply repellents to every exposed area of the skin. So imagine my surprise when I came across claims that a bee sting can actually be good for you, and, indeed, that the more you get, the better off you are. It seems that some people subject themselves to as many as 4,000 stings a year—twenty to forty per session three times a week! No, these are not masochists; they are people who suffer from osteoarthritis and rheumatoid arthritis, gout, acute sore throat, chronic headache, ongoing pain due to any cause, psoriasis, AIDS, and multiple sclerosis (MS). The most dramatic testimonials I have read are from MS patients. (The International Apiary Society, founded in 1983, is said to be keeping records of the effectiveness of bee venom in MS, and is following the progress of some 4,500 people with this disease. The Multiple Sclerosis Society takes the possibility of benefit seriously enough to have awarded a research grant to assess its effectiveness.)

The venom from the bee (delivered in its sting), and other bee-related products such as raw honey, propolis (a resinous substance from the leaves and bark of trees on which bees feed and which they then metabolize into a flavonoid-rich antioxidant), royal jelly, bee pollen (which isn't made by bees, but which they carry from flower to flower), and beeswax have been employed for medicinal purposes for centuries, and in China since antiquity. Their use is undergoing a resurgence in this country.

Despite the many publications in Asian and European literature documenting the safety and effectiveness of bee venom (in persons not allergic to it), there is a paucity of evidence in our own medical literature concerning its usefulness. In this country, bee venom therapy (BVT) is approved only to desensitize people who are dangerously allergic to bee venom and who could die from anaphylactic shock after being stung. (Everyone who is allergic to bee venom and who has not been desensitized should carry special syringes prefilled with adrenaline and "ready-to-go," although 95 percent of all allergic reactions to "bee sting" are actually caused not by bees but by wasps or yellow jackets.)

Bee venom contains several active substances, including the anti-inflammatory agents melittin (many times more potent than the steroid hydrocortisol) and adolapin. It also has an abundance of neurotransmitters such as dopamine, serotonin, norepinephrine, and histamine, all of which together not only make you shout "Ouch" but can also allegedly help reduce the severity of a variety of disorders. How they do so (if at all) is not clear, but, in addition to its obvious local effects, the bee sting is also thought by its proponents to "stimulate the immune system," a common, if vague, claim made by so many alternative practitioners. Everyone agrees that people with heart trouble, tuberculosis, diabetes, syphilis, gonorrhea, and women in the midst of their menstrual period should not take bee venom, even when it's given by injection under the skin rather than by a live sting, because of the shock and inflammation the sting provokes.

Doctors who can't arrange for a live bee sting can use bottled venom, although venom kept in a vial loses its potency. If your doctor approves it, you can also get apitherapy from specialized beekeepers. They'll remove the bee from a jar and apply it with tweezers to the desired area of your skin, which it then proceeds to sting. The stinger can either be removed immediately or allowed to remain for a few minutes. I have no idea how that decision is made. The usual number of stings per session ranges from two to five, although some gluttons for punishment have many more. Many people become adept at this themselves, keeping a jar of bees at home so they can perform the therapy on their own. (But always have an allergy workup before receiving this treatment to make sure you're not allergic to the venom.)

The American Apitherapy Society, with 1,600 members, estimates that there are 10,000 lay practitioners in this specialty. One physician alone, Dr. Christopher Kim of the Monmouth Pain Institute in Red Bank, New Jersey, claims to have given more than 3 million venom injections to 2,000 patients with a variety of pain syndromes.

❖ ❖ ❖　The bottom line? As you may have deduced, I am not "into" bee venom therapy, for two reasons: I'm not crazy about bee stings, and I could find no convincing evidence that it works. But if you're interested in learning more about the subject or how to get stung, write to the American Apitherapy Society, Inc., P. O. Box 54, Hartland Four Corners, VT 05049; telephone 800-823-3460.

❖ 9 ❖

BODYWORK

How Healing Is the Touch?

Except for a diagnostic push or poke, doctors don't usually touch their patients these days. In fact, it's unethical for psychologists and psychiatrists to have any physical contact whatsoever with their patients. But that wasn't always the case. Touching used to be the very foundation of the healing art. Centuries ago, for example, Hippocrates wrote a book on massage, and for many years massage was part of the medical school curriculum. Patients used to rate their doctors not only for their knowledge, personality, and diagnostic acumen, but also as masseurs. Then came all the machines, the miracle drugs, and the shortage of time (massage is so labor-intensive), and doctors began to delegate the body rub to others. So it's no longer a good idea to ask your doctor for a massage at your next visit. And in the unlikely event that he or she agrees to do it, don't expect your health insurance carrier to pay for it!

Nevertheless, when a doctor touches a patient, a bond is created between them. The touch sends a message that the physician cares. It was unthinkable for therapists in earlier times not to have such physical contact with their patients. That point of view has now been resurrected and has fostered a field known as "bodywork."

Bodywork ranges from simple touch to complicated massage and manipulation. Its goal is both psychological and physical improvement. As you will see, some bodywork methods make sense and have been shown to be effective; the evidence for others is less convincing.

Touch is perceived through myriad sensors in the skin connected not only to the brain but to other important organs as well. These sensors are designed to transmit different sensations; some are specific for light touch, others for deeper pressure, pain, heat, or cold. Their distribution varies too, so that some parts of the body are more responsive to a particular sensation than others. The feet, for example, are more sensitive than the hands, and the eye is infinitely more sensitive than the feet; our erogenous zones yield especially agreeable feelings. Strangely enough, the fingertips, so sensitive to touch, are less vulnerable to pain. These variations in sensitivity are important in terms what kind of hands-on treatment is employed, at what intensity, where, and why.

Shiatsu and acupressure (see chapter 4) and reflexology (see chapter 29)—widely used touch techniques—are referred to elsewhere in this book. In the following pages I will describe several types of bodywork that focus on movement, posture, and meditation. Although each has its own characteristics, their basic principles are identical.

The Alexander Technique

The Alexander technique was, believe it or not, devised at the turn of the century by a Shakespearean actor named

Frederick Matthias Alexander. It is now used by thousands of practitioners whose clients swear by it. Among its more notable adherents have been Aldous Huxley; John Dewey (who considered the technique so fundamental to learning, competence, and well-being that he recommended it be taught in all elementary schools); George Bernard Shaw; the Nobel Prize–winning scientist Nikolaas Tinbergen; and, more recently, Paul McCartney, Joel Grey, and John Houseman. Although their endorsements are hardly equivalent to scientific documentation in controlled studies, they are nevertheless intriguing.

The Alexander technique is a form of body therapy based on the premise that most of us don't have our heads screwed on properly. I'm perfectly serious! The goal of treatment is to correct the posture of the head, neck, and spine. Although some enthusiasts believe that this therapy can also improve a wide array of disorders such as asthma, ulcerative colitis, stomach ulcers, and high blood pressure, most practitioners recommend the Alexander technique as an effective aid to physical and psychological well-being—and nothing more. Specifically, they claim that it reduces back pain, eliminates learning blocks, and restores one's rapport with the environment.

You might wonder how it came about that this particular form of therapy was conceived by an actor. It is said that Alexander was having trouble projecting his voice to an audience. He had no problem with normal conversation, but as soon as he stepped onstage, his voice lost its usual power. When his doctors were unable to explain what was happening or to improve matters, Alexander tried to solve the problem himself. He spent hours emoting in front of a triple mirror and noted that this caused the muscles in his head, neck, and spine to go into spasm. He then spent the next few years devising a way to correct these postural abnormalities, and when he had devised it, his voice problem disappeared. Word of his success traveled like wildfire, first among his fellow thespians, and eventually throughout the world. The Alexander technique is currently most popular among dancers, singers, actors, musicians, and other performers.

From his initial aim—improving posture—Alexander evolved a much more ambitious goal and concept. Flushed with success, he began to attribute spiritual qualities to his technique, which he said applied to every religion. His concept of God was that of a "high power within the soul of man" that enhances, directs, or guides behavior. It is not clear to me how or why this spiritual aspect was invoked, or what it had to do with the mechanical interrelationship of the structures that disturbed Alexander's vocal cords. Other bodywork methods also claim to have a spiritual base, though, especially those originating in Eastern religions. Interestingly, most Alexander practitioners with whom I have discussed this aspect of their technique remain down-to-earth and focus on the physical basis of their manipulation.

The Alexander technique teaches normal upper-body posture—how to sit, walk, and stand—so that you can once more enjoy the physical flexibility of childhood. If you've forgotten what that was like, just watch any three- or four-year-old. As we age, according to the Alexander school, we are burdened with the baggage of muscle spasm, which distorts our normal anatomy. This happens so gradually and insidiously that few of us are ever aware of it. Alexander therapists have you "unlearn" this spasticity with a combination of exercise and gentle manipulation. In Alexander's words, "Change involves the carrying out of an activity against the habit of life." You are guided through a series of movements related to sitting, standing, walking, and talking. It's by no means a passive process, but one that requires your active participation through a combination of awareness and relaxation. Believe it or not, that's not an oxymoron.

❖ ❖ ❖ What's the bottom line? There is considerable anecdotal evidence, and many personal testimonials, that the Alexander technique does help. Persevering in it can improve posture, which can confer other benefits. Experiments at Tufts University in the 1970s showed that habitual responses that interfere with or impair normal function can be unlearned. So, should you sign up for an Alexander program? It certainly won't harm you, and it may very well help tension headaches, chronic neck and back pain, old whiplash injuries, and muscle spasm due to repetitive strain. But don't expect it to cure your asthma, ulcers, colitis, or gallstones.

Feldenkrais

Moshe Feldenkrais was a Russian-born physicist whose curriculum vitae would have appealed to Walter Mitty. Not only was Feldenkrais involved in nuclear radiation research and antisubmarine technology; he also introduced judo to the West and was one of the first Europeans to earn a black belt. He was a cartographer, a mechanical engineer, and an educator as well. How did he end up being a bodywork maven? Apparently, he injured his knees very badly and was left virtually crippled. He was determined to walk again, even though his doctors weren't able to restore full mobility. Searching for an answer, he began an exhaustive study of psychology, neurophysiology, physics, biology, and theories of learning, all of which he coordinated with his expertise in physics and Newtonian mechanics. He applied what he learned to body movement, and he succeeded in walking again. How he did this is embodied in the Feldenkrais method, which is now practiced worldwide.

This is a training program (Feldenkrais never considered it either a form of medical therapy, or even bodywork for that matter) to improve flexibility, coordination, range of motion, and function. Feldenkrais practitioners, unlike those of other forms of bodywork, make no exaggerated claims on its behalf. Although it is offered to people of all ages, both healthy and impaired, it appears to produce the most impressive results in people with neuromuscular disorders such as multiple sclerosis, cerebral palsy, and stroke. Some of the most enthusiastic reports are from older people who learn to move more easily and comfortably, with greater coordination.

The Feldenkrais method has two components—Awareness Through Movement (ATM, a copyrighted trademark) and Functional Integration (FI). Most participants start with the ATM sessions, movement lessons without a hands-on component. While you lie on your back on the floor, sit in a chair, or even stand, you focus on and feel the presence of various parts of your body and become acutely aware of them. As you meditate in this way, the instructor guides you verbally through a sequence of simple movements repeated several times. This process requires you to think, sense, and imagine as you go along. For example, you may be asked, "What is your left shoulder doing as you perform this movement? Is it tilting up or down, to the right or to the left?" By the time you have completed a few of these sessions, each of which usually lasts thirty to sixty minutes, the range of movement in the treated joints and muscles may be appreciably increased. There are hundreds of different movement lessons from which to choose, depending on your particular needs.

The Functional Integration aspect of the Feldenkrais method is a hands-on session. For FI, you lie on a table, sit, or stand. Again, you are guided through the same series of movements as in ATM, but this time an instructor gently manipulates your muscles and joints. This makes it possible for him or her to sense the resistance or compliance of your body as you perform each movement.

If the concept appeals to you, ask for a videotape from a Feldenkrais instructor in your area, call the Feldenkrais Guild at 303-449-5903, or write to the guild: P. O. Box 489, Albany, OR 97321. The guild has more than 1,000 members and some thirty training programs throughout the country. The Feldenkrais people take their mission seriously. Theirs is not a diploma mill, and accreditation requires three to four years of formal training.

❖ ❖ ❖   What's the bottom line? I am partial to most of these bodywork programs. Gentle ones like the Feldenkrais method can't conceivably do any harm. There have been several impressive reports of improved movement in normal subjects, the elderly, people with spinal injuries, and those with various motor problems.

Rolfing

Rolfing (Structural Integration), a variation of body manipulation, was developed by a biophysicist named Ida Rolf. Her technique differs from the others in that its focus is not on muscle and bone but on the connective tissue (fascia, the wrapping that binds and connects them). Strands of fascia come together at the end of the muscle to form a tendon, which in turn is what attaches muscle to bone. Normal fascia is loose, moist, and mobile, allowing muscles and joints to move easily and remain flexible. Chronic stress and inactivity cause the fascia to thicken and its layers to become glued together. That's what you feel when you have a "knot" in a muscle, usually in the back of the neck or in the chest wall. The body then tries to adapt by contracting the muscles and putting them into spasm. But that only makes matters worse, because it "freezes" the abnormal posture and interferes with the proper alignment of the head, trunk, pelvis, legs, and feet.

The purpose of Rolfing is to stretch and unwind the thickened fascia, reestablish proper alignment, restore the normal relationship between bones and muscles, and improve their function. Your friendly Rolfer applies sliding pressure to the involved areas—head, shoulder, chest, pelvis, and legs—with the thumbs, fingers, and sometimes even the elbows. Rolfers claim to be able to reduce pain and spasm, raise your energy level, improve your mood, and leave you more limber, with increased range of motion in your joints. The usual program consists of ten two-hour sessions one to two weeks apart. Each treatment builds on the previous one, so that the results of the therapy are said to be cumulative.

There are several hundred Rolf practitioners in the United States and throughout the world. The original Rolf Institute is in Boulder, Colorado, but there are at least two other schools in this country. Like many other bodywork techniques, this one takes itself seriously. To qualify as a therapist, you must have a bachelor's degree and then complete seven months of classroom work. After that, you need a license, requirements for which vary in different states.

Aside from personal testimonials, is there any hard proof that Rolfing works? Although pain cannot really be objectively measured, range of motion in a frozen joint can, and documentation of greater range of motion does exist, from a controlled study at UCLA's Department of Kinesiology. (Note that kinesiology is not to be confused with applied kinesiology, discussed in chapter 5.) Rolfing was found to have resulted in:

- Movements that were smoother, of greater range, and less constrained
- Fewer extraneous movements
- More dynamic and energetic body movements
- More erect carriage and less obvious strain to maintain a position

Studies at the University of Maryland reached similar conclusions. Other beneficial effects have been noted in children with cerebral palsy, and in persons with whiplash, chronic back pain, and curvature of the spine.

❖ ❖ ❖ What's the bottom line? Think of Rolfing as a physiotherapy program. If the program you're following isn't helping, it may be worth your while to give Rolfing a roll. (One of my neighbors is a Rolfer who loves to play golf. We call him Rolfer the golfer.) You can get the name of a local therapist from the Rolf Institute in Boulder.

Hellerwork

Hellerwork, an offshoot of Rolfing, was developed by Joseph Heller, an aerospace engineer at NASA. Heller became interested in humanistic psychology, gave up engineering, and was trained in Rolfing by Ida Rolf herself. He went on to become the first head of the Rolf Institute in 1976 but later introduced his own modification of this technique.

The objectives and techniques of Hellerwork are identical to those of Rolfing: greater mobility, and easier, painless body motion by means of hands-on manipulation. The difference is that Hellerwork includes a verbal dialogue to reduce emotional stress. The course consists of eleven sessions, each lasting forty-five minutes to one and a half hours, at a cost of $60 to $120 per session. One innovative technique is "before and after" videos that permit the client to see exactly which postural and other physical characteristics need changing, and how successfully he or she is progressing.

❖ ❖ ❖   What's the bottom line? It's the same as for any of the other bodywork programs. It's really a crapshoot which one will leave you more limber, relaxed, and pain-free. You may need to try more than one.

Trager

Trager (Tragerwork, Trager approach, Trager psychophysical integration) is a well-known and popular technique. I am fascinated by the different personalities and backgrounds of the innovators of these methods. We have already seen that one of them was a Shakespearean actor, another a nuclear scientist, and a third a biophysicist. Milton Trager was an M.D., an acrobat, and a boxing trainer. Soon after he became a doctor, Trager embraced the teachings of the Maharishi Mahesh Yogi, who brought Ayurvedic medicine to this country (see chapter 7). Trager was among the first eight American initiates; he focused on meditation therapy, which he later incorporated into the Trager method.

The Trager approach involves having your body rhythmically rocked, bounced, cradled, and moved by the therapist (there are now almost 10,000 Trager therapists) in order to loosen the joints, eliminate chronic tension, enhance relaxation, and increase range of movement. Each session lasts from sixty to ninety minutes, and you continue with them as long as necessary. Tragerwork is said to help persons with asthma, autism, polio, muscular dystrophy, multiple sclerosis, and a variety of other neuromuscular disorders. Coupled with this physical approach is Mentastics, a form of mental gymnastics which Dr. Trager also believed could retard the aging process.

Proof? Mostly anecdotal case histories of improvement of chronic pain, and better muscular function after polio, spinal cord injuries, multiple sclerosis, cerebral palsy, and other such disorders.

❖ ❖ ❖   What's the bottom line? The same as for other bodywork programs. In my view, they all have a potential to improve muscle function. View them as an extension of physiotherapy. If your present regimen isn't working, one of the above may, but don't expect to be cured of any diseases.

Yoga

Yoga is something everybody has heard about but few people really understand. To most of us, it conjures up visions of swamis, gurus, and other exotic Eastern holy men; or visions of people standing on their heads or sitting immobile in Buddhaesque positions. But that's not the yoga that is used in many rehabilitation centers, Veterans Administration hospitals, by physiotherapists, or indeed, anywhere the crippled and disabled are treated. Some of my own colleagues who practice traditional medicine recommend yoga to patients with neuromuscular disorders.

Yoga has no religious connotations for most of those who use, enjoy, and benefit from it. Simply stated, it is a technique with three major components: posture, breathing, and meditation. Its purpose is to strengthen and relax the body. Admittedly, though, much of what I found in the Indian literature on the subject, which dates back thousands of years, is mumbo jumbo to my Western mind.

In a typical yoga class, you perform various physical exercises in which you assume certain postures. (Eastern literature contains delicious descriptions of these positions—the grasshopper, the cat, the bee, etc.) There are eighty-four different postures (called *asanas*), of which five are the most important. (Their names are jawbreakers, so I won't list them here. What? You insist on knowing them? Okay. They are *padmasana, bhadrasana, virasana, vajrasana,* and *svastikasana.* I warned you.) The first objective of yoga is to maintain one of these poses for varying periods of time, and that's not easy. It takes considerable training and discipline to do it right. Your yogi (as a yoga teacher is called) suggests the best posture for you and teaches you how to do it. Although the immediate purpose of mastering these postures is to improve the circulation, stimulate the abdominal organs, stretch the body, and restore the normal alignment of its various structures, its ultimate purpose is the self-control needed for proper breathing (*pranayama*) and for effective meditation (*pratyahara*). The breathing exercises consist of a routine in which the breath is "stretched"—the lungs are filled with air which is held and then released—all in a prescribed manner. Learn to do that, and you'll find the meditation part easier.

Meditation detaches you from your environment; your goal is to avoid experiencing any emotions or feelings while meditating. If you do it right, meditation allows you to enjoy the kind of deep concentration that can lead to "peace, enlightenment, and tranquillity." Some yogis also use incantations and magic, but these have not really caught on in this country. There are unsubstantiated reports of yogis who bury themselves alive or remain underwater for days, or stand on one foot for years. They believe that such strenuous training demands and encourages spiritual growth and a balanced mind. I haven't met any of them and don't recommend that you seek them out. Stick to the exercises, the breathing program, and meditation.

Here is a scaled-down version of yoga that you can follow easily and effectively, as described in the University of Texas–Houston *Lifetime Health Letter* of January 1996:

- *For exercise:* Sit forward in a chair, your feet flat on the floor. Put your right hand on your left knee. With your left hand, hold the back of the chair. Look straight ahead, inhale, and then as you slowly exhale, turn to your left. Pull with both hands to rotate your spine as much as possible without strain. Hold the rotated position for a few seconds, continuing to breathe easily. Return to the forward position. Then put your left hand on your right knee, and repeat the steps, twisting to the right.
- *For breathing:* Sit straight with both hands flat against your stomach, just below the navel. Relax your stomach and allow it to push out as you inhale. Then, as you exhale, tighten your stomach and flatten your back. Concentrate on the sound your breath makes in the back of your throat. Breathe smoothly and steadily through your nose; don't hold your breath at any time. Repeat this procedure several times.
- *For meditation:* Sit quietly and comfortably in a chair or on the floor. Close your eyes and take a few full, deep breaths. Concentrate on the sound you make when you breathe in and out. Relax your breath, and at the same time, consciously relax your facial muscles. Progressively relax the rest of your body, beginning with the shoulders and arms, working your way down to your feet. Become limp without slouching. Try to be completely silent, inside and out. Imagine a pleasant scene to help yourself achieve total relaxation. After a few minutes, begin to breathe more deeply; then stretch your arms and imagine your energy being totally renewed.

Several scientific reports suggest that yoga can reduce blood pressure and heart rate, improve circulation, and enhance memory. Some of these benefits may be due to a release of endorphins, the natural opiates produced by the brain—the mechanism also invoked to explain the effects of acupuncture (see chapter 4).

❖ ❖ ❖ What's the bottom line? The people I know who practice yoga love it. Does it cure any disease? I doubt it. Does it relax you, bring equanimity, or ease chronic pain? Probably. Will it improve your memory? Possibly, if it teaches you to concentrate better. Should you try it? If you're so disposed; but you may have trouble finding a good yoga instructor, because there are no certification standards or programs. I suggest you contact the International Association of Yoga Therapists (109 Hillside Avenue, Mill Valley, CA 94941; telephone 415-383-4587) for the name of a yogi in your neck of the woods.

Prolotherapy

Prolotherapy (sclerotherapy), another variation on the body-works theme, is specifically directed to the treatment of back pain. Americans searching for relief of back pain spend at least $20 billion a year on physiotherapists, acupuncturists, chiropractors, orthopedists, osteopaths, and other therapists. Every single day in this country, it is said, one person in five suffers an acute attack of back pain.

Prevailing wisdom among most "back mavens" is that back pain is almost always due to a "slipped disk," degenerative arthritis of the spine, or simply muscle spasm. The usual "establishment" therapy consists of anti-inflammatory drugs, cortisone shots, or surgery. Bodywork enthusiasts employ a combination of manipulation and relaxation techniques. But according to prolotherapists, the main cause of the problem is not disease of the spinal bones or nerves, but *instability* of the vertebrae that constitute the spinal column. They point out that if you X-ray most people after age fifty or so, you can see arthritic changes and narrowing disk space in their spines, even if they have no symptoms. In the prolotherapists' view, the ligaments, whose function is to maintain the normal alignment of the spine, are the main culprits. As we get older, these ligaments stretch, becoming lax and weak, and causing the spinal column to wobble all over the place. Muscles in the area go into spasm to provide some stability, and it's the spasm that causes the pain. But since muscles alone cannot provide the necessary stability, prolotherapists direct their therapy at the ligaments.

Prolotherapy involves no exercise, surgery, or medication. Instead, the therapist injects an irritant solution into the affected area of the back. This is a variation of the sclerotherapy used in the conventional treatment of varicose veins, in which a chemical injected into a dilated vein causes it to scar and close. In prolotherapy, this irritant solution allegedly attracts blood cells called macrophages; these are scavenger cells which then remove the irritant solution. When they've finished, they leave the scene and are replaced by fibroblasts, whose job is to repair the damage in the area. The fibroblasts do this by laying down scar tissue that reinforces the weakened ligaments. Prolotherapists claim that this enhances the strength of these ligaments, which are then able to align the spine properly, eliminate pain, and restore mobility. They claim a success rate of 92 percent and further assert that there is no downside to this treatment. They promise permanent cure of chronic back pain after ten to fifteen treatments, each of which costs between $100 and $200.

Prolotherapy has been described in scientific medical journals such as *The Lancet,* as well as in osteopathic publications, but it is not endorsed or widely used by conventional physicians. Prolotherapy is on the fringes of chiropractic and osteopathy, and I could find no convincing scientific evidence that it works. If you're interested in learning more about it, contact the American Association of Orthopedic Medicine, 435 North Michigan Avenue, Suite 1717, Chicago, IL 60611; telephone 800-992-2063.

Polarity Therapy

Polarity therapy falls somewhere between therapeutic touch and magnetic therapy (see chapter 25). The concept was developed in the early 1900s by Randolph Stone, a chiropractor, osteopath, and naturopath. He believed that the human body is an electromagnet, surrounded by a magnetic field. In his view, the pulsating energy that makes up this field consists of specific frequencies of life energy from such elements as "ether, air, fire, water, and earth." In order to function in a state of good health, the atoms in this field must be properly aligned. Stress, injury, and exposure to powerful electromagnetic fields in our environment all cause the normal orientation of the atoms to go askew, resulting in many of our physical and emotional symptoms.

Polarity therapists claim to correct this problem by transferring biomagnetic energy from their own hands to their clients' bodies, relaxing the tissues and muscles and improving circulation and well-being. In addition, they provide nutritional guidance, teach gentle stretching exercises, correct any misalignment of the spine, and offer "polarity verbal guidance" whose purpose is to create "life-enhancing thought."

I view polarity therapy as a variant of bodyworks, one that can provide soothing massage. Although several books have been published by its practitioners, I was unable to find any references to it in the scientific literature. As with many other bodywork techniques, I do not give credence to the grander health claims, but if you find the massage relaxing, go ahead and treat yourself to it.

Prayer and Mental Healing

I am not really qualified to discuss prayer and mental healing, phenomena that medical science cannot explain. There have been reports of healing, cures, and spontaneous remissions resulting from prayer and faith accompanied by the laying on of hands—and even without direct touch. Skeptics ridicule these reports, saying that all such events are either fabricated, hysterical, inaccurate, or based on misdiagnosis. Frankly, I have never met a true "healer" (other than a good doctor) or seen any kind of distant healing (by prayer or voodoo). However, I am not prepared to say categorically that it cannot occur. I never discourage anyone who has the kind of "faith" that leads him or her to seek spiritual or mental healing. If it works for you, go for it. I don't recommend that you pursue it in place of conventional therapy, but I see no reason not to include it as part of your treatment.

❖ 10 ❖

CELL THERAPY

Who Sells These Cells—
and Should You Buy Them?

What did Winston Churchill, Pope Pius XII, Emperor Hirohito, Dwight D. Eisenhower, Charles de Gaulle, Aristotle Onassis, a potpourri of royalty (including the Windsors), and scores of celebrities (all quite rich) have in common? They were all injected, at a clinic in Switzerland, with cells (or extracts)—live, freeze-dried, or ultrafiltrated—from animal organs or embryos. And many of them said that they had thereby discovered a fountain of youth! Thousands of people continue to be intrigued by the premises and promises of cell therapy: the hope of "rejuvenation"; the prevention or cure of cancer; a strong immune system; sexual vitality; no more arthritis; less heart disease; an easier menopause; and the successful management of painful menstruation, infertility, herpes, chronic bronchitis, premature aging, epilepsy, and mental retardation. In short, there's a promise of something for everyone in cell therapy. But you do need thousands of dollars to pay for it. If you plan to try cell therapy, bring plenty of cash. No third-party payer that I know of will reimburse you.

Therapy with animal cells (usually from sheep) is popular in Europe, where it was introduced, as well as in Nassau, Mexico, and several other places. However, it is not approved or practiced in the United States.

Paul Niehans, a Swiss physician, pioneered sheep-cell transplantation. Here is what led him to believe it could be effective in treating a wide variety of ailments. In 1931, in the midst of an operation on a woman's thyroid gland, the patient's parathyroid glands were inadvertently damaged. These tiny structures, situated very close to the thyroid, produce a hormone that controls the level of calcium in the blood. When it drops too much, as it did in this patient's case, convulsions set in. There was no time to transplant a fresh parathyroid gland from a steer calf, as Niehans had planned to do, so he hurriedly mashed the animal's parathyroid tissue in a salt solution and injected it into the patient. Her convulsions stopped, and apparently she had normal parathyroid function for the rest her life.

This dramatic experience suggested to Niehans that cell transplants, rather than whole-tissue or organ transplants, from healthy animals might benefit a patient with a weak or otherwise deficient organ. This is not implausible. After all, we were already transfusing blood cells by the 1930s, and we are now performing transplants of bone marrow, which also consists of cells. One difference, however, is that these are human-to-human transfers, not transplants between species.

Initially, Niehans extracted live cells from specific organs of freshly slaughtered sheep and injected these cells directly into patients. This raised the specter of infection, because to be viable the cells had to be injected immediately after being harvested, and there really wasn't enough time to make sure that the donor animal was completely healthy. Another problem was rejection of this foreign tissue by the host (the patient). At that time, Nestlé, a Swiss company, had just developed the freeze-drying technique for coffee, and Niehans adapted it to his cell transfers. Now he was able to freeze-dry fresh cells, sterilize them, and store them for several weeks, if necessary, before injecting them. This did not solve all his problems; for one thing, the surface of frozen cells still contained enough active protein to cause rejection. The next step was the development of a technique of ultrafiltration that removed most of this protein but left enough cellular components to be effective. Niehans believed that these cells stimulated and enhanced the function of their human counterpart organs. And there you have the theory and the rationale behind cell therapy.

Currently, clinics providing this therapy use cells from a wide range of animal tissues such as sex glands (for which I am told there is great demand), parathyroid, adrenal, liver, pituitary (the master gland in the brain), and others. The most frequent source of these cells is still sheep, although pigs have become increasingly popular because their cells are more like those of humans.

Injected cells are "organ-specific": that is, adrenals go to adrenals, kidneys to kidneys, gonads to gonads, liver to liver, and so on. When the host tissue—the patient's own tissue— is weak or wanting, these infusions are said to perk it up. Having trouble urinating? I've got just the sheep kidney for you! Impotent? How about some extra pig testicle? There's a shot for virtually every tissue or organ in the body. Can't you just see these cells, injected into a human's bloodstream, scattering in every direction, making a beeline for the host's counterparts?

The proponents of cell therapy also believe that it stimulates the entire immune system, not just specific organs. So if you feel lousy all over and can't put your finger on what ails you, you are given total embryo shots, all mashed up. These allegedly contain everything you might possibly need. Two to five injections of the total embryo extract will do the trick.

Frankly, I find it hard to believe any of this, in the absence of any scientific documentation. But it's easy to see how appealing this simplistic concept might be to someone with problems that conventional medicine can't solve.

Peter Stephan, a doctor who operates a clinic on Harley Street in London, has come up with a variation of Niehans's cellular therapy. Instead of injecting cells directly into his patients, he first gives them to another mammal, which responds by making antibodies (antibodies are part of the body's immune system). When there are enough of these antibodies in the second animal's bloodstream, they are removed, further purified, and *then* given to the patient, very much like a vaccine. Stephan claims that this technique effectively boosts the human immune system and has no side effects.

Cellular therapy in one form or another has been claimed to be effective against arteriosclerosis, Down's syndrome, Parkinson's disease, hepatitis, skin conditions, and a host of other disorders. In my opinion, none of the evidence offered for these claims has satisfied the criteria demanded by the scientific community, however. "Proof" usually takes the form of a testimonial by a patient or a statement from a doctor that goes something like this: "This man had no sex drive at all, but after a course of these injections, he was indefatigable." "This woman had severe hepatitis and after only three or four shots, she was cured." No less a luminary than the heart surgeon Christiaan Barnard extolled the virtues of cell therapy. He cited as "proof," without any other documentation, his own response to arthritis-specific cell therapy. I'm not disparaging such testimonials or denying their sincerity, but they're simply not enough to allow the conclusion that cell therapy, as currently administered, is effective.

Can cell therapy prolong life or improve its quality? Not according to any of my own patients who've been to these clinics, or anyone else I know. The only effect they describe, thousands of dollars later, is a sore arm at the site of the injection.

Even though I was unable to find any documentation in the scientific literature for the claims made in behalf of cell therapy, I decided to include it in this book to make sure that you do not confuse these treatments with the promising human fetal cell transplant programs currently under way in this country. The cell therapy provided at Clinique La Prairie in Switzerland, the International Clinic for Biological Regeneration in England and the Bahamas, Stephan's clinic in London, and other commercial facilities has nothing to do with the research being conducted with human fetal tissue for such disorders as Parkinson's disease, Alzheimer's disease, and diabetes.

❖ ❖ ❖ The bottom line? In the near future, species-specific cells—from human to human—may help patients with Parkinson's disease or other neurological conditions, diabetes, or even heart problems (through replacement of cardiac cells damaged by heart attacks). However, I cannot at the present time recommend the cell therapy of Niehans and his disciples.

❖ 11 ❖

CHELATION
Magic Bullet—or Bull?

Patients are always asking me about chelation. They have heard, usually from a friend, that it unblocks clogged arteries everywhere in the body. Should they try it? How does it work? What will it cost? Is it dangerous? Will their insurer reimburse them for it? Here are the answers to these questions.

The term "chelation" is derived from the Greek word *chele,* meaning "claw." The concept of chelation is based on the observation that when a certain amino acid complex, ethylenediamine tetraacetic acid (mercifully abbreviated EDTA), comes into contact with certain positively charged metals and other substances such as lead, iron, copper, calcium, magnesium, zinc, plutonium, and manganese, it grabs them (hence the "claw"), and removes them. Chelation is the standard, accepted, and best way to treat heavy-metal poisoning, including the lead poisoning that threatens the lives of so many children. Injected into a vein, EDTA hunts down the harmful metal and combines with it, and both are then excreted from the body through the kidneys. Used in this way, EDTA has saved many lives since it was first synthesized in 1930.

So what's the controversy? About forty years ago, noting that EDTA was being used by plumbers to remove calcium from pipes and boilers, some doctors speculated that it might do the same for arteriosclerotic—"hardened"—arteries, where plaques (thickened patches containing cholesterol, some calcium, and other substances) obstruct the flow of blood. They tested their hypothesis by feeding rabbits a high-fat, high-cholesterol diet long enough to produce arteriosclerosis in the animals' blood vessels. When they injected them with EDTA, the plaques melted away! The doctors concluded that what's good for rabbits must be good for people, and began using EDTA to treat patients who had obstructed blood vessels.

Thousands of doctors now chelate some 500,000 people every year in this country alone. They have established their own professional societies with such names as American Academy of Medical Preventics (I couldn't find the word "preventics" in my dictionary), American Board of Chelation Therapy, American College for Advancement in Medicine, and American Holistic Medical Association. They contend that chelation is the most effective and most economical way to prevent and treat blood vessel disease—as well as Alzheimer's, complications of diabetes, and a host of degenerative disorders for which conventional medicine has relatively little to offer—and to slow the aging process. In their view, bypass surgery, angioplasty, atherectomy and endarterectomy (in which obstructing arterial plaques are scraped away) are unnecessary, expensive, and dangerous. These procedures, they argue, generate billions of dollars for hospitals, cardiologists, and a vast support staff of care providers, which is why mainstream medicine continues to use them and persistently rejects chelation. The "establishment," on the other hand—the FDA, National Institutes of Health, American Medical Association, American College of Physicians, American Heart Association, American Academy of Family Physicians, American Society of Clinical Pharmacology and Therapeutics, and American Osteopathic Association, to name a few—asserts that chelation is unproven, ineffective, dangerous, and expensive, and that its practitioners are money-hungry charlatans.

Who's right? Let's first look at the validity of the theoretical claims for and against chelation, and then examine the evidence relating to its effectiveness.

Most doctors believe that the rationale for treating arteriosclerosis with chelation is flawed. They point out that most of the calcium removed from the body by EDTA comes not from blocked arteries, which contain very little, but from bone—its richest source in the body. They also explain that even if EDTA did remove some of the tiny amounts of calcium in arterial walls, this would make very little, if any, difference to the flow of blood. That's because the major constituents of the obstructing plaque are scar tissue, cholesterol, blood cells, fibrin, and other substances—not calcium. The small amount of calcium present is deposited late in the course of arteriosclerosis, moreover; and thus it is not an important contributor to enlargement of plaque or to arterial obstruction by plaque. Finally, the decrease in plaque size after EDTA therapy, induced experimentally in rabbits, has never yet been demonstrated in living humans. So the theory that chelation increases blood flow by shrinking arterial plaques doesn't hold water, as far as they are concerned.

◆ ◆ ◆

Theoretical considerations aside, is there any proof or even any evidence that chelation works? The scientific community is swayed by facts, not testimonials. Before prescribing and administering EDTA to their patients, doctors would like to see convincing data from double-blind experiments on large numbers of patients (see chapter 2). They expect chelation to meet the same rigid standards required by the FDA before it approves any drug or treatment as "safe and effective." What's the track record so far?

In reviewing the available medical literature on the subject of chelation, I found no proof that it affects any disease process one way or another. The many claims for relief of symptoms were difficult to interpret because of so many confounding factors. For example, in one study, in addition to injecting their patients with EDTA, the doctors also got them to adopt other healthful measures; they made them stop smoking, lose weight, exercise regularly, and take vitamin supplements, all of which can have an impact on the way someone feels. So who can tell if the EDTA did anything? I came across a report of 153 persons who had pain in the calf of the leg when walking because their leg arteries were diseased. The study was double-blind, all the patients were assigned randomly either to control or to treatment (with EDTA) groups, and blood flow in the diseased limbs was measured before and after chelation therapy. Although both the placebo and the chelation groups reported improvement in symptoms, there was no objective, measurable difference in the blood flow within their arteries after six months of treatment.

This is very much like what I have occasionally seen in my own practice. I'm not suggesting that the following two cases are statistically significant, nor do I offer them as proof, one way or another, about chelation. However, they do illustrate how difficult it can be to assess the significance of a clinical response that is not documented objectively. One of my patients, a fifty-eight-year-old diabetic man, had severe disease of the arteries in his legs. Doppler (sound wave) studies revealed an 80 percent narrowing of a large artery in one leg and a 90 percent obstruction in the other. There are no conventional drugs that will dissolve these plaques or significantly improve the blood flow through them. The best that any doctor can do for such a patient, short of surgery, is to try to get him or her to stop smoking (this man didn't smoke) and encourage exercise to stimulate a collateral circulation—the gradual opening up of new arteries when the native arteries are diseased. I gave my patient what advice I could. After an absence of three years, he showed up again. He told me that he had resorted to chelation "in desperation," because my regimen hadn't helped him. And now—whereas he had once been able to walk for only two blocks before the pain set in—he could go at a reasonable pace for ten blocks. He was impressed—and so was I! However, when I repeated the Doppler studies, I found the same obstructions that had been there before the chelation! Why was he feeling so much better? I'm not sure. It wasn't because chelation had shrunk his plaques. Perhaps the EDTA had in some way affected the muscle metabolism in his legs so that the muscles were able to make do with less blood flow, or perhaps he had developed a more effective collateral circulation during the interval, independent of the chelation. Or was it all a placebo effect (see chapter 2)? Your guess is as good as mine.

The second patient, also male, had severe angina, the chest pain that signals heart disease. I arranged for him to have a coronary angiogram to see if he was a candidate for bypass surgery. Unfortunately, he was not. Although his arteries were very diseased, they were too small to accept a graft of a new, clean artery or vein. So I treated him with every available medication. He did improve somewhat—but not enough to suit him, and at the suggestion of a friend, he decided to try chelation. He was a no-show at my office for a few months. When he did come back to see me, though, his angina was much improved. (He had also continued the medication I originally prescribed.) I was eager to evaluate the status of his coronary artery disease objectively and had him perform a treadmill test. (In this procedure, the patient walks on a treadmill at a given speed on a specific incline. We then see how long it takes before chest pain sets in, and at what point the electrocardiogram becomes abnormal.) This man had taken such a test before his chelation, so I was interested to see whether there was any objective evidence of his subjective improvement. Here is what I observed. He developed the very same ECG changes he had shown before chelation, and at the very same point in his exercise. The only difference was that this time he had no pain. I stopped the test when the ECG abnormalities appeared, and don't know how long he would have been able to continue before developing pain. Again, I cannot explain why he felt no pain, since the same ECG abnormalities appeared.

The chelationists' reply to all this is that the negative scientific studies in the mainstream literature were all done by hostile researchers, that the chelation wasn't administered properly, and that they, the chelationists, have in fact proved the efficacy of this treatment. They point to the 3,569 abstracts submitted to the American Academy for Advancement in Medicine by its members. In his book *Bypassing Bypass* (Hampton Roads, 1990), Elmer Cranston claims to have reviewed more than 4,600 documentary reports in support of chelation therapy. I found that the great majority of these papers rely more heavily on anecdotes than on science. However, a handful did contain positive, supportive data.

◆ ◆ ◆

Where do we go from here? First, let me say that I do not believe that practitioners of chelation are, as a group, dishonest or exploitative. Those whom I know personally are convinced of its benefits. Many take this treatment themselves and give it to their families and friends. But it's unfortunate that they accuse the skeptics of conspiring to withhold an important advance from the American public for personal gain. The truth is there's more potential income to be had from chelation than from most conventional cardiac procedures. A course of chelation therapy consists of twenty to thirty intravenous injections, one to three a week, each lasting about three and a half hours. The customary charge is about $100 per session. This adds up to a total cost of approximately $3,000. (The cost of an uncomplicated bypass usually runs between $20,000 and $30,000.)

I have been speculating about other mechanisms that might explain the beneficial effects claimed for chelation. Here's one that appears to make sense. The villain in arteriosclerosis is LDL, the "bad" form of cholesterol. (HDL is the "good" or protective component.) LDL circulating in the bloodstream is sucked into the wall of the arteries, where it stimulates chemical changes that lead to the formation of arteriosclerotic plaques. This harmful process is aggravated by free radicals in the area—end products of oxygen metabolism in the body. (Free radicals are analogous to the exhaust of a car. They cause all kinds of bad things, including this effect on LDL in the arterial wall.) That's fact, not theory. Where does chelation enter the picture? Free radicals need metals, especially copper, in order to do their dirty work with the LDL. By removing copper from the area, EDTA may conceivably have a beneficial effect. Binding iron in the same way may also help. Is the action of EDTA on calcium a red herring? Probably not, because calcium ions in the lining of the arterial wall and its cells may contribute to a thickening of the wall, and their removal may possibly slow down the arteriosclerotic process. So it's the effect of chelation on the free-floating calcium, not the hardened stuff in the plaques, that we should be looking at.

This theorizing about the beneficial action of EDTA is plausible, but the battle lines have been so rigidly drawn that any conventional doctor who even considers such ideas publicly risks incurring the wrath, or—worse—the contempt of his or her colleagues. My own position is that, given the fact that 1 million Americans die every year from cardiovascular disease, it's the duty of the scientific community to evaluate chelation seriously, thoroughly, and definitively. If we're not happy with how the chelationists gather and interpret their data, let's formulate and fund the kind of research with which everyone will agree—and get on with it. The FDA had planned to conduct such studies, but I understand they were canceled because of lack of funding. Someone should do them.

❖ ❖ ❖ So what's the bottom line? At the moment, there is no real proof that chelation works, but there are some appealing theories that suggest why it may work. Is it dangerous, as is still alleged by some people? Years ago there were reports that chelation disturbed cardiac rhythm, damaged the kidneys, and could even cause death. However, the new, lower doses of EDTA now being given appear to be safe. In a large study acceptable to proponents and critics alike, EDTA administered according to the current guidelines was found to be no more toxic than a placebo.

What should *you* do, pending the results of definitive research, if you have a significant disability or symptoms? Go the conventional route first. Despite the attacks on bypass surgery and other interventions, they are at present the best treatment for obstructive disease of the blood vessels and can be lifesaving. But if you are not a suitable candidate for bypass, angioplasty, or any of the other conventional techniques, and medication is not helping as much as you'd like, try chelation. There may be something to it. To find the right doctor to perform it safely, write the American Board of Chelation Therapy, 70 West Huron Street, Chicago, IL 60610; telephone 312-266-7246.

❖ 12 ❖

CHIROPRACTIC
A Disjointed Theory?

Back pain is the most common cause of disability among Americans under the age of forty-five; 80 percent of us experience an acute "back attack" some time before our fiftieth birthday. The annual cost of managing back disorders in this country is about $25 billion. Most people treat a "bad back" with aspirin, Tylenol (acetaminophen), or nonsteroidal anti-inflammatory agents such as ibuprofen and naproxen. They go to bed with a heating pad or an ice pack for a day or two, then get up, go back to work, and hope for the best. During the first forty-eight hours after a "back attack," I suggest you use an ice pack for ten minutes several times a day; after that, hot baths, showers, and a heating pad are more effective.

If this do-it-yourself approach doesn't work, and the pain is severe or recurrent or becomes chronic, the next step is a visit to a "health care provider." (Remember when this person was called a doctor?) The "provider" may be a primary caregiver, a family doctor, an orthopedist, a physical therapist, a physiatrist, an acupuncturist, a masseur or masseuse, an osteopath—or, for one in three patients, a chiropractor. Patients ask me almost every day which one is best. If you've been agonizing over this decision, remember that in nine out of ten adults, the acute problem subsides on its own within four weeks, *regardless* of whom you see or what he or she does for you. If you consult your *family doctor,* he or she will usually send you to bed (unnecessarily, in most cases) and prescribe painkillers (okay as long as you keep taking them) and cold or heat applications. That's what you'd have done anyway, $25 or $50 earlier. If you go to an *orthopedist,* either on your own or because your doctor has referred you, the action escalates and the costs go up. You will almost certainly be asked to have back X rays, which usually turn out to be normal. If you don't have a herniated disk or some other condition that may require surgery, the orthopedist is likely to send you to a *physiotherapist.* You can now expect several exercise sessions—on dry land or in a pool—to limber up your tight muscles. You also may be given local electrical stimulation or may be referred to a *physiatrist* (basically a physiotherapist with an M.D. degree) for Novocain, saline, or alcohol injections of your "trigger points" (bundles of muscle fibers that have gone into spasm and are often responsible for the symptoms). Should you decide on *acupuncture* (because "everyone" is doing it these days), an attempt will be made to restore your *yin-yang* balance with needles inserted into specific sites in your body, often far removed from the back itself (see chapter 4). An *osteopath* manipulates not only the spine but other parts of the body as well. And then there is the *chiropractor.* What is a chiropractor, and if you're in agony should you see one right off the bat?

• ◆ •

The bitter fight between chiropractors and "real" doctors began years ago—and it continues to this day, though perhaps with somewhat less animus. The School of Chiropractic was founded near the end of the nineteenth century by a "magnetic healer" named Daniel David Palmer. Canadian by birth, Palmer moved to Davenport, Iowa, where, as a young man, he raised bees, sold raspberries, and ran a grocery store. He became interested in osteopathy and magnetic healing. Magnetic "therapy," in which the patient's body is stroked so as to increase its "magnetic flow," was then practiced by many lay healers and some physicians. Palmer learned the technique and opened an office in Iowa in the 1880s. One day in 1895, in the course of a visit for some complaint or other, a janitor in his office building told Palmer that seventeen years earlier, after he had strained his back, his ears had "popped"; he became deaf and had remained so ever since. In the course of examining this man's spine, Palmer found one of the vertebrae to be displaced. He manipulated it back into its normal position and the patient's hearing was restored! That's how chiropractic was born!

Palmer reasoned that improper alignment of the spine presses on nerves that leave the spinal column at various levels to supply virtually every organ in the body. This disrupts the normal flow of nerve impulses and interferes with normal muscle function, respiration, heartbeat, arterial tone, digestion, and resistance to disease. According to Palmer, correcting the alignment—which he called "chiropractic," meaning "done by hand"—would release the pressure on the nerves and restore health. He emphasized that the vertebral column is not a rigid structure that houses and protects the nerves coming from the brain, but a series of twenty-four joints, each of which must be intact and flexible. He believed that virtually every disease, not only back pain, is due to slippage—he called it "subluxation"—of one or more of these bones. In his view, the treatment of every health problem requires correcting subluxation. He taught these theories at the Palmer Infirmary and Chiropractic Institute, which he founded in 1897, and from which the first fifteen chiropractors (five of whom were physicians) graduated five years later. Among the graduates was his son, Joshua, who would carry the chiropractic torch for the next fifty years.

There have since been many variations in the techniques of chiropractic. There are currently three basic categories of practitioners: "straights," "mixers," and the rest. The "straights" remain convinced of Palmer's original concept, that virtually every illness—infection, arthritis, high blood pressure, heart attack, you name it—is due to subluxation. They not only correct these slippages when you are sick; they also recommend that you get your spine checked regularly in order to stay healthy. The "mixers," who outnumber the "straights," also focus on maintaining the mechanical integrity of the nervous system, but they concede that there are other causes of illness, such as bacteria. In addition to correcting your subluxations, "mixers" will also advise you about nutrition and lifestyle; give you a therapeutic massage, or ultrasound, or even an enema now and then; and perform a variety of other holistic measures. Chiropractors in the third, as yet unnamed, category have a more limited point of view. They restrict their therapy to nonsurgical neuromusculoskeletal disorders (pain due to muscle spasm, nerve inflammation, or bone problems such as arthritis) and make no claims about curing the gamut of diseases targeted by the "straights." There are additional subspecialties within these different areas of chiropractic, each of which focuses on its own special technique.

There are some 50,000 licensed chiropractors in this country, who deal with millions of office visits a year. Chiropractic is the fourth largest health profession—after physicians, dentists, and nurses.

As noted above, there is an ongoing controversy between chiropractors and medical doctors. Most orthopedists and osteopaths deny that there is any such thing as subluxation. Although mechanical derangement of the spine does occur, they say it is not universal, as claimed by chiropractors. The medical profession considers subluxation to be more of a chiropractic state of mind than a physical abnormality of the spine. Despite the long, rigorous formal education (usually some four years at an accredited institution) required of chiropractors before they can be licensed, the medical establishment views them as tradesmen with scientific pretensions, and some M.D.s rankle when chiropractors call themselves "doctor."

In recent years, however, chiropractors have successfully fought for recognition as providers of legitimate medical therapy, especially for back pain. Government bodies at various levels have granted them licensure; at least half of the insurance companies now pay for chiropractic treatment; a recent law in Florida allows members of HMOs to see a chiropractor for diagnosis without a referral from a primary care doctor; and some hospitals have given chiropractors staff appointments, although they must care for their patients jointly with a physician. These changes have taken place because several studies have shown that chiropractic treatment of low back pain is at least as effective as ministrations by doctors of medicine—and usually less costly.

A comprehensive review by the Agency for Health Care Policy and Research (AHCPR) and the U.S. Department of Health and Human Services (USDHHS) determined that "spinal manipulation is recommended and efficacious for at least the first month for acute low back pain problems in the adult." This report criticized the habit—almost a reflex— that many doctors have of ordering expensive tests, such as X rays, CT scans, and magnetic resonance imaging (MRI), before trying manipulation, even when there is no suspicion of a fracture, a tumor, infection, or severe nerve involve- ment—all relatively uncommon. The study concluded that manipulation should be tried before resorting to surgery (which is needed by only one in a hundred people with acute low back pain); and that spinal traction, biofeedback, trans- cutaneous electrical stimulation, acupuncture, and injec- tions are virtually useless. (I heartily disagree.) The study also denounced the use of drugs, steroids, antidepressants, "disorienting painkillers," and extended bed rest, none of which is used by chiropractors.

Another study—the Manga report, in 1994, commissioned by the Ontario Ministry of Health—goes even further. Its authors also conclude that in treating acute back pain, chi- ropractors are at least as effective as doctors—and less costly—and that chiropractors should therefore be the pri- mary caregivers for such patients.

On the other hand, the most recent study of the relative merits of the various forms of therapy—this one conducted by the North Carolina Back Pain Project and involving almost 1,600 patients—concluded that patients with acute low back pain have similar outcomes whether they are treated by primary care practitioners, chiropractors, or orthopedic surgeons. Moreover, this study found that "pri- mary care practitioners provide the least expensive care for low back pain." The average number of back-related visits was 3.1 for HMO doctors, 5.5 for orthopedists, and 15 for chi- ropractors. The typical bill for a primary care doctor with an HMO was $435; $746 for an orthopedist; and the typical bill for the chiropractor's sessions was $783, presumably because a chiropractor has you come back more often and for a longer period of time. Nevertheless, in this study patients expressed the greatest satisfaction with the treatment provided by chiropractors, even though the long-term outcome was no different. They found the chiropractors' examinations more thorough and their explanations more reassuring. It is clear that the chiropractor, whatever else he or she does, spends more time with the patient, generally shows greater interest, and is more apt to discuss *all* of the patient's symptoms, not just the back pain itself.

Is there a role for chiropractic for symptoms other than low back pain? There may be, according to a representative sampling of published scientific reports that suggest that chiropractic may be helpful for:

- Bed-wetting in childhood
- Duodenal ulcers
- Dysfunctional uterine bleeding associated with low back pain
- Facial muscles affected by Bell's palsy
- Erb's palsy (a limp arm due to pressure on the nerve supplying it) in infancy
- Diabetic polyneuropathy presumably worsened by malfunction of the muscles and joints of the foot
- Shoulder pain
- Carpal tunnel syndrome
- Herniated disks in the cervical spine (neck)
- Electric shock (which has damaged the muscular and nervous systems)
- Headaches due to poor alignment of the cervical spine
- Pregnancy (among 170 pregnant women with back pain, those who received chiropractic manipulation of the spine had significantly fewer symptoms)

However, you should also be aware of some negative reports about chiropractic. There have been instances of life-threatening dissection (tearing) of a major artery to the brain during spinal manipulation. If you have any blood vessel problem, check with your doctor before allowing a chiropractor to perform such manipulation. Manipulation of the lower spine can also lead to complications such as bladder disturbance, leg weakness, and rectal and genital malfunction.

Such reports highlight the importance of choosing a chiropractor as carefully as you would select any other health provider. Check with your local or state chiropractic society for a list of accredited practitioners.

❖ ❖ ❖ The bottom line? If you suddenly develop a bad back, and you're not helped by aspirin, Tylenol, or one of the over-the-counter nonsteroidals such as Aleve or Advil; and if you've also tried cold or heat—then you may consult any of a variety of health care providers. In the long run, none is likely to help you more than any other.

I sometimes refer my patients with back pain to a chiropractor, though not to one of the "straights" or "mixers." I emphasize to the patient that there is no credible evidence that chiropractic does anything for AIDS, pneumonia, a heart attack, or any other illness. If you are referred to a chiropractor, check on the credentials, make sure he or she is licensed, and ask your doctor to discuss your case with him or her before your visit. Quite frankly, if there is any question about diagnosis, I prefer an osteopath to a chiropractor, if I can find one who still focuses on manipulation. An osteopath is permitted to prescribe any medication that may also be necessary in addition to whatever manipulation he or she performs. A chiropractor is not. Also, if your back pain happens to be due to a serious underlying cause—such as a cancer that has spread to the bone, or a collapsed vertebra due to osteoporosis—a good osteopath is more likely to make the diagnosis than a chiropractor. These complications are relatively uncommon, especially in younger persons, but they do occur. I expect that chiropractors will bridle at these statements, but that's been my experience over the years.

❖ 13 ❖

CRANIOSACRAL THERAPY

Heads You Win.
Tails You Win, Too?

I had never even heard of craniosacral therapy before I started writing this book. However, when I looked into it, I was surprised at the number of people who not only knew about this therapy but had actually received it at some time or another. The usual reason was to relieve chronic headache. It was my impression that most of them felt better after the treatments, although not for very long. Virtually every doctor with whom I discussed craniosacral therapy, including several neurologists, knew very little about it and didn't care to know more.

Here is how craniosacral therapy is said to work. Cerebrospinal fluid (the stuff doctors remove when they stick a needle into your back to do a spinal tap) bathes the brain and the tissues of the spinal cord. It is prevented from leaking out into the rest of the body by a membrane (the meninges) that encloses the entire nervous system. (Inflammation of this tissue envelope around the brain is called meningitis; in the area of the spinal cord, it's referred to as spinal meningitis.) Cerebrospinal fluid normally flows freely from the head (cranium) to the base of the spine (sacrum). According to craniosacral therapists, this nervous system circulation has a rhythm of its own, as does the circulatory system. They theorize that anything that interrupts the normal flow of the cerebrospinal fluid, or alters its rhythm and pressure, can cause physical and mental problems. So far so good—sort of. But here's where they lose me. Craniosacral therapists claim that when they run their fingers lightly over the bones of the skull, or anywhere along the spinal column, they can actually feel the flow of this fluid. If it seems abnormal to them, then, by applying gentle massage and pressure, they can correct whatever is awry— and relieve a variety of symptoms. That, in short, is what craniosacral therapy is all about.

Unfortunately, none of my colleagues in the everyday world of medicine—among others, some very good neurologists—has ever seen, touched, or had any other contact with cerebrospinal fluid except after withdrawing it for analysis. This fluid is not palpable in an adult. It is true that during infancy the bones of the skull are made of relatively soft cartilage and are separated by suture lines; but these bones harden and fuse as we grow older, covering the meninges. Run your fingers over the top of your own head. Do you feel any gaps, fluid waves, or pulses? I can't, and although I have a full head of hair, I doubt that I could even if I were bald.

Proponents of craniosacral therapy insist that the suture lines present at birth never close completely, and that they actually move slightly in response to changes in pressure in the spinal fluid. It's along these patent suture lines that the trained cranial therapist claims to be able to detect, evaluate, and if necessary "correct" the flow of the cerebrospinal fluid. However, in my view, if the suture lines remained open, you would expect them to "give" when someone sustained a fracture of the skull, but they almost never do.

Everyone agrees, however, that in infancy the bones of the skull are mobile before they close; and it is in the very young that craniosacral therapists report their greatest successes. The conditions that are said to respond best during infancy are earaches, hyperactivity, vomiting, irritability, and sinus congestion, all of which are believed to be due to injury and compression of the base of the skull during the birth process. Adults with migraine headaches, chronic neck and back pain, depression, anxiety, sciatica, trauma from automobile or other accidents, dyslexia, and even Down's syndrome are said also to benefit from craniosacral therapy. A course consists of three sessions, costing between $50 and $150.

William Sutherland, an osteopath, formulated the theory of craniosacral therapy in the early 1900s. During the last twenty years, his work has been continued and popularized by another osteopathic physician, John Upledger. In the late 1970s, Upledger headed a team of scientists at Michigan State University who produced a model demonstrating the movement of fluid in the nervous system from the head to the sacrum (tailbone). They concluded that the craniosacral system acts like a semiclosed hydraulic system. I understand this to mean that within the system, a certain amount of "give" is possible: that is, the membranes surrounding the cerebrospinal fluid are able to fluctuate. Anything that interferes with spinal fluid flow prevents this "give" and raises the pressure on the membranes as well as the tissues of the brain or the spinal cord, resulting in pain from your head to your tail, as well as emotional and behavioral problems.

Although there are innumerable testimonials from patients to the effectiveness of craniosacral therapy in the treatment of chronic headache and other symptoms, there is little if any substantiation in the scientific literature. For example, there was a recent study of twelve patients—children and adults—all of whom had some condition for which craniosacral therapy is alleged to be effective: physical trauma, surgery, learning disability, etc. Craniosacral motion and fluid pressures were analyzed in each subject by three different craniosacral therapists, who failed to agree on the findings in any of the cases.

❖ ❖ ❖ What's the bottom line? There are ongoing studies to see whether any of the claims for craniosacral therapy can be validated. In my own opinion, the laying on of hands—as, for example, in massage or shiatsu—can relieve symptoms of tension, especially in the area of the head and neck. To the extent that craniosacral therapy involves such contact, it can help. On the basis of the available evidence, however, I do not buy the theory about fluid movement and manipulation. Despite support by such respected figures as Dr. Andrew Weil, who reports anecdotally on successes achieved by one of his friends who is a craniosacral practitioner, I am not recommending this therapy to my own patients. By the same token, though, I am not discouraging anyone for whom conventional treatment has failed from trying it, since it can do no harm.

❖ 14 ❖

DIET THERAPY FOR CANCER

Does What You Eat
Really Make a Difference—Now?

One of my friends used to be a heavy cigarette smoker. Although she was persuaded to quit, and hasn't touched a cigarette in years, she still hankers after the weed. When we're sitting together near someone who is smoking, she discreetly leans into the stream of secondhand smoke. She tells me, perfectly frankly, that although she has no intention of ever smoking again, if she were to develop cancer, she would immediately light up. At that point, she says, there would no longer be any reason to abstain. She also feels the same way about a "healthy" diet; she'd go right back to fat and cholesterol if she developed a malignancy. Would you?

There is no question that over a lifetime, you will reduce your chances of developing cancer if your diet is high in fiber and low in fat (especially from animal sources) and includes lots of fruit, vegetables, and whole grains; and if you go easy on alcohol, and foods that have been salt-cured, salt-pickled, barbecued, or smoked. But does it make any difference what you eat *after* you have cancer, especially once the cancer has spread? Should you now throw caution to the winds, eat whatever you like, and let the devil take the hindmost?

The "establishment" response to these questions is mixed. You will find the most up-to-date "official" position in Dr. Daniel Nixon's excellent book, *The Cancer Recovery Eating Plan* (Times Books, 1996). Individual oncologists may be nihilistic about diet after cancer has struck, but nutritional scientists are not. They feel strongly that what you eat is important not only *before* you have cancer, but also when there is a premalignant tumor such as a bowel polyp, leuko-plakia (white plaques that often become cancerous, com-monly seen on the tongue of a heavy smoker), and even when cancer is already present but hasn't spread. Under all these circumstances, eating much more fiber and much less fat can reduce the chance that a cancer-causing agent will damage cellular DNA, and can stop the cancer-enhancing activity of abnormal genes. So if you have an early cancer, consult a nutritional scientist for specific nutritional advice. The vari-ous regimens he or she can offer are well described in Dr. Nixon's book. However, even the most enthusiastic nutri-tionally oriented establishment specialist will tell you that no dietary regimen makes a significant difference once a cancer has spread, or metastasized.

It is at this point that conventional and complementary medicine part company. In this section, you will read about several alternative dietary regimens for the management of "terminal" cancer, their rationale, and whether there are any data to justify their use. Decide for yourself whether they are worth trying. But when comparing any of these alternative approaches with traditional methods, remember that traditional treatments can rarely cure a cancer that has already spread. Given this poor track record, I find it hard to understand the arrogance of the "establishment" in deprecating complementary approaches born of desperation. It's one thing to caution against using an unproved treatment instead of a conventional treatment that works, but it's ludicrous to attack an unproved treatment without offering a better option. That's saying, in effect, "Your program doesn't work; neither does mine. However, I'm a scientifically trained doctor and you're not. So it's okay for me, but not for you, to administer useless toxic agents."

Someone who is dying and desperate is not concerned with turf wars or credentials. That's why more and more people with terminal illnesses are turning to complementary techniques, even though there is little statistical proof that most of them are effective. Such patients have little to lose. Can you blame them for exploring every avenue? Let me, however, reemphasize that *cancer can often be cured by conventional methods if it is found early enough.* Do not even look at any of the alternatives described in the following pages until you and your doctor are absolutely certain that your cancer has spread and that the mainstream treatment you're receiving is an act of futility.

Most conventional doctors lose interest in encouraging you to make lifestyle changes once you have cancer (unless, of course, it's skin cancer—in which event you'll be warned to stay out of the sun). Their focus now is on surgery, radiation, and chemotherapy. Some physicians don't even bother to have you quit smoking if you have lung cancer at this "late stage," even if it was probably caused by cigarettes in the first place. They go along with any change in your eating habits that makes you happy. Since most patients with advanced cancer are poorly nourished anyway, the usual objective is to try to get as many calories into you as possible—by mouth, tube, or vein. It's assumed that calories from any source strengthen the immune system and help cancer patients withstand the stress of chemotherapy. So almost every physician I know (like the traditional Jewish mother) encourages his or her cancer patients to eat, eat, eat and rejects any dietary restrictions that could result in further weight loss. However, this assumption has never been proved. In fact, total parenteral nutrition (hyperalimentation)—administering massive amounts of calories intravenously—has not been shown to make one iota of difference to the survival of patients with advanced cancers, and in fact may even be harmful.

There has been a backlash among members of the alternative medicine community against this "let them eat cake" attitude. They point out that, statistically, the more affluent the society and the more calories it consumes, the higher the incidence of cancer. This is most evident in hormone-related tumors such as those involving the prostate, breast, colon, and ovary, as well as in leukemia and rectal cancer. According to the American Cancer Society, overweight men are at 50 percent higher risk of developing cancer. In laboratory experiments, animals who have lost significant amounts of weight after being deprived of food, especially protein, are less susceptible to certain cancers. Tumors that have been experimentally produced or transplanted into them grow more slowly. However, when these animals resume their usual diet, their cancers thrive. These observations suggest that cancer patients should be *underfed,* denied certain foods, and made to *lose* weight in order to "starve" the tumor, and that overfeeding nourishes cancer cells and helps them spread. It has even been proposed that cancer patients should not have supplements, such as folic acid, pyridoxine, or riboflavin. Withholding them presumably hurts cancer cells more than normal cells.

Several nutritional regimens for treating cancer are based on these concepts. Some appear to make sense; others, however, are bizarre. Although no dietary regimen I know has ever cured cancer, some can improve the patient's outlook or otherwise have a positive effect on the quality of life. Oddly enough, it's the most stringent and punishing diets that seem, at least anecdotally, to have the greatest effect.

The dietary regimens discussed below vary considerably: one has you eating only raw food; another insists that everything be cooked; you may be required to eat only organic foods or restrict your protein intake; you may have to push potassium or cut down on salt; you may be permitted to continue "conventional" anticancer therapy or ordered to discontinue it. Despite their differences, however, these nutritional regimens are almost all basically vegetarian, low in fat, and high in fiber—very much like what the establishment is recommending for *prevention* of cancer, or the management of early growths that remain contained.

Many patients with cancer feel instinctively that food must play some role in its causation, but they hesitate to follow any diet that has not been proven effective or is ridiculed by their mainstream doctors. But with the clock ticking away, what choice do they have? If you are in this quandary— or if someone you love is—the following descriptions of nutritional regimens may help you make a decision.

Wheatgrass Diet

Wheatgrass is the early form in the growth of a variety of plants that ultimately become grains. The earliest anti-cancer diet on record is the wheatgrass regimen, recommended by Hippocrates (whose oath your doctor took when he or she graduated from medical school). His modern disciples, led by Ann Wigmore (who died in 1994), have set up wheatgrass treatment and education centers throughout the world. There are three in this country, one of which is the Ann Wigmore Institute (now run by Shu Chan). Despite her interest in nutrition and cancer, Wigmore's only degree from an accredited school was a doctorate of divinity.

The curative powers of wheatgrass, upon which cattle everywhere graze, were the focus of Wigmore's fascination. She became enthusiastic about wheatgrass after observing that dogs, cats, and other animals nibble on grass when they're ill and seem to feel better afterward. Her speculation about the benefits of wheatgrass were reinforced by the biblical account of Nebuchadnezzar, the king of Babylon. He is said to have lived in the wilderness for seven years, apparently insane, eating grass and living like an animal. But he recovered spontaneously presumably due to the healing powers of the grass. (Another interpretation of the same account, however, has it that Nebuchadnezzar was banished by the deity and sentenced to wander in the wilds for seven years because of his arrogance. He was scheduled to be rehabilitated after that time, wheatgrass or no.) In any event, Wigmore concluded that enzymes in raw wheatgrass were "alive" and could detoxify an intestine poisoned by rotting food. According to her, chlorophyll, which she referred to as the "lifeblood of the planet," is the major therapeutic ingredient in wheatgrass. Wigmore emphasized that to benefit from wheatgrass, it must be juiced and consumed fresh.

Wigmore's followers claim that the wheatgrass diet stimulates the immune system, kills harmful bacteria in the digestive system, and eliminates wastes and toxins from the body. How it does all this is not clear, nor have the toxins it is said to help the body excrete ever been identified, by Hippocrates or anyone else. Other key aspects of the original Hippocratic diet are restriction to "live" food—juices, nuts, seeds, fruit, and sprouts, supplemented by a variety of enzymes and green algae. None of this may be cooked—and don't even think about eating any meat, dairy products, or fish. Lifestyle changes, details of which are described in publications by the wheatgrass centers (available at health food and other stores), are promoted in the wheatgrass clinics. Prominent among them are regular "detoxification" by enemas and high colonics (see chapter 18).

I have heard testimonials from cancer patients that the wheatgrass diet either cured their cancer or slowed its progress, but I have found no credible, objective evidence to substantiate a single one of these reports. On the other hand, there are many accounts of *adverse* reactions from the wheatgrass regimen.

❖ ❖ ❖   Here's the bottom line concerning the wheatgrass diet. If you have cancer, and simply hate cooked food, meat, dairy products, and fish, but are nuts about nuts, seeds, raw vegetables and sprouts, all washed down with wheatgrass juice, and if you're prepared to subsist totally on such a menu, go for it. But to do it the "right" way—the Wigmore way—you'll also have to be detoxified on a regular basis with lots of enemas and high colonics. If you decide to follow the wheatgrass diet, get plenty of vitamin supplements, especially B_{12}, and don't you dare abandon any other conventional treatment recommended by your establishment doctor. Always remember, too, that enemas involve a risk of infection and perforation of the bowel.

Macrobiotic Diet

The macrobiotic diet doesn't have the ancient pedigree of the wheatgrass regimen, but it is now the most widely followed alternative nutritional program in this country. It has many variations, depending on who's prescribing it, where, and for what reasons. The most popular macrobiotic diet consists of 50 to 60 percent whole-grain cereals, 20 to 25 percent vegetables, 5 to 10 percent beans and sea vegetables (nori, wakame, kombu, dulse), and 5 percent soups. No macrobiotic diet includes meat or poultry (thus this regimen leaves you vulnerable to vitamin B_{12} deficiency). Here's the rest of what's forbidden: eggs and dairy products; animal fat; refined sugar; tropical or semitropical fruits; carbonated beverages; artificial drinks; caffeine or aromatic teas; food that's been colored, treated with preservatives, sprayed, or subjected to pesticides and other chemicals; refined and polished grains and flours; any canned, frozen, or irradiated foods; hot spices—and alcohol. You eat complex carbohydrates; the higher the fiber content and the less saturated the fat, the better; vitamins and minerals should come from natural food sources, not supplements; sea salt, not table salt, is used for seasoning; all food is organically grown, unrefined, and never chemically treated; vegetable protein is preferred to animal protein; food is cooked over gas or in a wood-burning stove, not by microwave or in an electric oven.

My wife and I, unabashed gourmets, had a recent experience with the macrobiotic diet. We were looking for a housekeeper-cook, and among the applicants was a very nice woman who seemed to fit the bill. We began the usual negotiations—salary, days off, benefits, and so on, and then got down to a deeper discussion of her cooking experience. What did she do best? What were her favorite dishes? That's when she dropped the bombshell! She proudly announced that she'd been following a macrobiotic diet for some time now and, personally, would eat nothing else. Her last employer was an elderly woman with cancer for whom a macrobiotic diet had been prescribed. Since it was too much work to prepare two separate menus, our potential cook tried this diet too, became accustomed to it, and felt infinitely better on it. She was also convinced that it had prolonged the life of her employer. Since she very much wanted this job with us, she was prepared to cook anything we asked for, as long as we would allow her to continue a macrobiotic diet for herself. She assured us that she would do so unobtrusively, without complicating our lives. And, by the way, were we at all interested in trying this diet ourselves, since "everyone" who follows it feels so "great"? Given my open mind on these matters, I asked her exactly what that would entail. What foods would we be eating, and what would we have to give up? She basically repeated the list described above. When I complained that it didn't seem very exciting, especially for a dinner party, she insisted that there was plenty of choice. For example, we could have cooked, organically grown whole-cereal grains such as barley, millet, rye, wheat, corn, and buckwheat (and she knew where to buy them). She could also prepare some nice whole-wheat pasta, and even bake whole-grain bread (without yeast, of course). There were several delicious soups on her menu, too, made with vegetables, seaweed, grains, or beans, seasoned to taste with soy sauce or miso. They'd do wonders for us, she said. The list of vegetables, organically grown, was virtually endless. We could have broccoli, cauliflower, bok choy (which I happen to love), scallions, onions, turnips, all kinds of squash, carrots, and several others, in unlimited quantities. However, iceberg lettuce, mushrooms, celery, cucumbers, snow peas, and string beans were permissible only in limited quantities. Unfortunately, potatoes, tomatoes, asparagus, eggplant, peppers, zucchini, spinach, beets, and avocados—all of which happen to be among my favorite foods—were entirely off-limits. But (and her face lit up when she told us this) we could have "some" different kinds of beans, many of which I had never even heard of— wakame, hiziki, kombi, and arame. I thought she was pulling my leg until she added the more familiar chickpea and lentil.

Our prospective cook (now not so prospective) sensed that we weren't exactly salivating at the prospect of dining at home in the future. My wife and I exchanged glances which asked, in effect, why we should go this spartan route, given that we were not suffering from cancer or any other illness. Being perceptive and possibly fearing that she wouldn't get the job, the applicant made a concession. Okay, she would stretch our macrobiotic diet to include small amounts of fish such as herring, scrod, snapper, halibut, and trout a couple of times a week. She also assured us that we would soon develop a taste for nonaromatic and nonstimulating teas such as roasted brown tea, bancha twig tea, and stem tea (none of which I had ever even heard of, let alone tasted). If we preferred the flavor of coffee, she knew how to make a delicious brew from cereal grain. Her own favorite beverage, she added, was plain water, not iced.

My wife and I were very impressed with the enthusiasm of our applicant—let's call her Ms. V.—and with her energy and her expertise with the macrobiotic diet. However, we explained to her that, since we were both relatively healthy, we saw no need to change our eating habits so drastically at this time, even though we were sure we would probably benefit from doing so. She took our dissent in stride. She would accept the position on our terms. We hired her.

Ms. V. turned out to be an excellent chef. She prepared our favorite courses for us—barbecued chicken, a steak now and then, some mouthwatering salmon, and even an occasional scoop of ice cream. For the first few weeks, she herself ate only a macrobiotic diet. Initially, there may have been a touch of disdain in her attitude toward our "gluttony." But then we began to notice that there were fewer and fewer leftovers in the fridge. For example, we couldn't find the ice cream we had saved for another repast; and some meat that could have been reheated the next day, or given to the dogs, had also disappeared. We suddenly realized that Ms. V.'s resolve had weakened. After a month, she came out of the closet and abandoned her macrobiotic diet completely. The epitome of tact, I never commented about it to her.

So now everyone at our home eats the same fare—and enjoys it. This is Ms. V.'s third year with us. We've all put on some weight but are otherwise very happy. Ms. V. makes, partakes of, and enjoys delicious roast chicken and curried snapper, and she mixes a mean martini to boot! Her current philosophy is that if she should ever develop cancer, that will be time enough for her to return to her macrobiotic diet.

Here's what I learned about the macrobiotic diet from Ms. V.'s experience: it's not hard to follow if you're committed to it, but it's easy to abandon when you're tempted and lack the motivation to continue. Unfortunately, the episode taught me nothing about its impact on cancer.

There are several clinics and centers here and abroad that offer instruction in macrobiotics. It's more than just a diet; it's a way of life. It originated in Eastern, especially Japanese, culture, not as a specific cancer preventive or treatment, but as a lifestyle whose goals are to enhance spiritual and physical well-being and to promote a philosophy of peace among nations. As stated by the Kushi Macrobiotic Institute in Massachusetts, a well-known macrobiotic center, its aim is to "provide the education necessary to achieve our common goal of a healthy and peaceful world."

Macrobiotics came to be used as a cancer treatment because its proponents are convinced that malignancy is the end stage of prolonged exposure to dietary and environmental toxins, a "wrong" outlook on life, and a sedentary existence. They believe that the main dietary nemeses are refined sugar and animal protein, but that any of the following can also cause a serious imbalance in our internal environment: milk; cheese; eggs; fatty or oily dishes; and anything that freezes or cools the interior of the body, such as a cold beer, cold fruit juice, a cold soft drink, a dish of ice cream, or a glass of ice water.

The cornerstone of this macrobiotic philosophy is a 4,000-year-old cosmologic theory, according to which everything in life relates to the relative proportions of *yin* and *yang. Yin* is centripetal (seeking the center); *yang* is centrifugal (moving away from the center). When your body is in perfect *yin-yang* balance, you enjoy "harmony" and health. Different foods are predominantly either *yin* or *yang;* so are different cancers. Cancers situated peripherally, and in the breast, are *yin* malignancies associated with too much sugar, spices, and citrus fruits. *Yang* cancers are said to be caused by animal foods and involve organs deep in the body, such as the colon. So the dietary management of a particular cancer depends on its type. *Yang* foods are emphasized in dealing with *yin* cancers, and vice versa. Once you've decided on the appropriate diet, you must chew each mouthful 50 times if you're healthy, and 150 times if you have cancer; this is to make sure that you don't eat too much.

The dietary differences between a macrobiotic regimen and what conventional oncologists recommend are obvious. The conventional diet is designed for the individual patient's immediate nutritional needs and preferences; the macrobiotic diet is rigid and restrictive. Mainstream doctors advise you to eat fats because they are calorically dense and low in bulk, and so they "go further" when you have no taste for food to begin with; macrobiotic diets, by contrast, are high in bulk and low in fat. A conventional doctor is likely to emphasize simple sugars for a quick "energy fix"; the macrobiotic school does not. Animal protein, as in milk and eggs, is the mainstay of the conventional cancer diet; by contrast, the macrobiotic diet focuses almost exclusively on plant protein.

Does a macrobiotic regimen permit you to continue your conventional anticancer therapy? Not really. You're generally advised to gradually taper off chemotherapy and other interventions. You are warned that unless you do, your recovery will be much slower. Various macrobiotic institutes and clinics claim that they've obtained the best results in people with cancers of the breast, cervix, colon, pancreas, liver, bone, and skin. Those with cancers of the lung, ovaries, or testes don't do as well. (The last two are eminently responsive to and frequently curable by conventional methods. I would *not* rely solely on any diet or unconventional approach in dealing with ovarian or testicular cancer.)

So much for the definition of the macrobiotic diet. Has its effectiveness been documented? The American Cancer Society (ACS) analyzed data submitted by the Kushi Macrobiotic Institute and found no evidence that the macrobiotic diet plays any role whatsoever in the prevention or treatment of cancer. What's more, in the opinion of ACS, this diet constitutes a serious hazard to health. The Office of Technology Assessment of the U.S. Department of Commerce has also reviewed the available literature on the subject. Most of what it found was anecdotal. Its analysts were unable to document or attribute to the macrobiotic diet any of the miraculous cures or salutary effects attested to by cancer patients and their families. In many of these cases, individuals following such a diet were also receiving conventional therapy, making it difficult to be sure what was doing what. Then there is always the question of the accuracy of the original diagnosis. Did all these patients really have cancer? For example, macrobiotic instructors have been known to label as "cancer" harmless swellings or discolorations on the upper bridge of the nose, blisters on the eyelids, or a blue-gray discoloration in the white of the eyes. However, in one study, thirty-six patients with cancer of the pancreas who followed a macrobiotic diet survived an average of six months as compared with a median national survival of three months. The problem with this research is that it was not randomized, so we can't separate any effects of treatment from the health profiles of the subjects. There are many potentially confounding factors in cancer of the pancreas that make it difficult to compare results in a highly selected group of patients with some unspecified "national" average. The same investigators also claimed that patients with prostate cancer who followed a macrobiotic regimen lived significantly longer than those on conventional regimens. A doctor named Anthony Statelier wrote a book entitled *Physician, Heal Thyself,* in which he recounts why he is convinced that a macrobiotic diet prolonged his survival after he developed prostate cancer (he died seven years later). The significance of his testimonial is weakened by the fact that prostate cancer can be very slow-growing, and survival for seven years is not unusual.

Not everyone who follows a macrobiotic diet has cancer. Ms. V. is a case in point. Many people are converted to it because it promises better health. If you look back at Ms. V.'s description of the macrobiotic diet, you see that because it permits so little fat and oil, it has fewer calories than are recommended by the Food and Nutrition Board (1,800 to 2,000 calories daily for women and 2,400–2,700 calories for men). Since most of the protein is of vegetable origin, it may lack certain essential amino acids. While it's true that you can add amino acids, the macrobiotic school does not encourage you to do so.

Some enthusiasts put their children on a macrobiotic diet too. That's not a good idea. Study after study has demonstrated that while several vegetarian diets are suitable for older children, macrobiotic diets are dangerous for children below the age of two years. Infants fed a high-fiber diet without any milk develop rickets, scurvy, anemia, and osteoporosis; the breast milk of "macrobiotic" mothers who consume little or no dairy products and meat contains less calcium, magnesium, protein, zinc, saturated fatty acids, and vitamin B_{12}. (A deficiency of B_{12} results in neurological problems, gastrointestinal disorders, and anemia in adults as well as children.) Every doctor with whom I have ever discussed this matter feels very strongly that mothers who are committed to a macrobiotic diet should be certain to provide their infants with additional fat (a minimum of 20 to 25 grams a day—1 tablespoon of any oil contains 15 grams; 1 teaspoon of butter has 5 grams), fish (100 to 150 grams per week—that's 3.5 to 5.5 ounces), and at least 150 to 250 grams of dairy products daily (4 ounces of cottage cheese contain about 110 grams). Older kids on macrobiotic diets are often undernourished, grow more slowly, have below-average psychomotor development, and have a variety of nutritional deficiencies. Pregnant women who follow a strict macrobiotic diet can become deficient in calcium and vitamins B_{12} and D—not good for mother or fetus. For all these reasons, the Council on Foods and Nutrition of the AMA and the Committee on Nutrition of the American Academy of Pediatrics have condemned the macrobiotic diet.

Despite all these criticisms by the scientific community, I believe that there should be a large trial—randomized, well documented, and with excellent record keeping—to determine whether, and to what extent, a macrobiotic diet, *properly supplemented,* prolongs survival in cancer patients or improves the quality of their lives.

❖ ❖ ❖   Until then, here's the bottom line:

• If you're pregnant and following a macrobiotic diet for whatever reason, take multivitamin supplements; make sure they contain vitamins B_{12} and D, and calcium; and get your obstetrician's approval that it is safe to continue the diet for the duration.

- Do not feed infants or children a macrobiotic diet without supplemental milk and fish, or without a pediatrician's supervision.
- Do not abandon any proven treatment for cancer in favor of a macrobiotic diet, especially if you're already undernourished. However, if you're determined to follow such a diet, make sure a qualified nutritionist attests to its adequacy.
- Although it is theoretically possible that a macrobiotic diet has a protective effect against some cancers by reacting in some favorable way with the body's hormones, this belief remains largely a matter of speculation.

The Gerson Diet

The Gerson diet is the prototype of some twenty "metabolic" anticancer diets currently in vogue. I'm not quite sure what the term "metabolic diet" means, but it usually embraces two concepts: "detoxifying" the body and "stimulating" the immune system. The Gerson diet is not nearly as old as the wheatgrass diet of Hippocrates, or as widely used as the macrobiotic diet.

Max Gerson was born and educated in Germany and practiced medicine there before coming to the United States in 1936 to escape the Nazis. An avid student, extremely intelligent, innovative, and of the highest personal integrity (I know all this from my nurse of many years, who worked with him until he retired), he built a successful practice in internal medicine in New York City. Gerson had many original and unique ideas about cancer and nutrition. He was convinced that cancer—along with several other "degenerative" diseases such as arthritis, multiple sclerosis, and diabetes—is caused by a breakdown of the immune system and other defense mechanisms. He thought this was the result of the American lifestyle, especially what we eat, because of the way our food is grown and processed (theories similar to those offered by the macrobiotic school). He blamed chemical fertilizers and pesticides that had left our grains, fruits, and vegetables with too little potassium and too much sodium, an imbalance aggravated by cooking and further processing. He postulated that these pollutants also poison the liver, leaving us more vulnerable to cancer. In his view, the only way to cure cancer was to correct these abnormalities. He proposed draconian measures, many of which are still followed at a clinic in Tijuana, Mexico.

What is the Gerson program? Does it work? Is it feasible? Has it met reasonable scientific standards of proof of efficacy?

Anyone who intends to follow the Gerson regimen should know that it is a full-time job and not for the fainthearted or those who live alone. Although Gerson's original program has been modified somewhat over the years, his basic formula is unchanged. For example, for the first four weeks of therapy, you must drink eight ounces of fruit and vegetable juice every hour for thirteen hours every single day. The juice must be freshly prepared every hour in a stainless steel grinder and press (centrifugal juicers and liquefiers are unacceptable because they are thought to destroy some of the enzymes). All this requires about 150 pounds of fresh organic produce a week. Originally, three glasses of juice from pressed raw calves' liver were also prescribed, but that requirement was discontinued after several patients became sick because of infected calves' liver. Potassium is added to every glass of fruit and vegetable juice. You must also have "three full vegetarian meals prepared from organically grown vegetables, fruits, and whole grains." That means, say, salad, baked potatoes, cooked and raw vegetables and fruit, and oatmeal. You need two tablespoons of linseed oil daily as well. Nothing you consume may come into contact with aluminum pots or pans.

The list of forbidden foods is very long. You may not have any animal protein (dairy products, meat, poultry, or fish) for the first four weeks, and may never again enjoy berries, nuts, salt, oil, coffee, or any food that's been bottled, canned, refined, preserved, or frozen. (And you thought the macrobiotic diet was tough?)

You can see why, what with all the pressing, squeezing, and shopping for fresh fruits and vegetables, someone following the Gerson regimen must have full-time live-in assistance. An administrator at the Gerson clinic is said to have estimated that it takes as much as fifty hours a week just to buy all the food, prepare it, and get the juices ready in the prescribed manner. That's a tall order for a healthy person, let alone someone debilitated by cancer.

But wait! There's more—much more. You must also take five grains of thyroid hormone. Supplemental thyroid hormone makes the heart beat faster and can also cause disturbances of rhythm even in persons with normal thyroid function. (I am particularly worried about its effect on the cardiac rate in someone with palpitations.) You also are given a solution of potassium iodide; six capsules of acidophilus pepsin; fifteen tablets of pancreatin (a digestive enzyme); royal jelly (a vitamin- and protein-rich extract of bee pollen); 300 milligrams of niacin; and periodic injections of vitamin B_{12} combined with crude liver extract. You must also stop all other medication you may have been taking, but you are permitted one aspirin tablet a day to relieve a headache or other mild pain.

Just reading about this regimen wears me out—and remember, I'm healthy! And we're not done yet; the best is yet to come. Toxins must be purged from your body, especially those hiding out in the liver. Early in the therapy, you will be given three to five coffee enemas every day, each one consisting of a dilute one-quart solution, sometimes supplemented with castor oil. These are supposed to stimulate the flow of bile, which allegedly carries "poisons" from the liver to the bowel, whence they are eliminated.

The Gerson clinic is now run by Gerson's daughter, among others. This new team is constantly adding to and modifying the program. For example, they may give you any or all of the following: ozone (usually by enema) or hydrogen peroxide (by a variety of routes; see chapter 28) "to destroy infections and promote normal healing"; an intravenous drip containing a mixture of potassium, glucose, and insulin; "live cell therapy" (see chapter 10); castor oil; clay packs; various vaccines, including one against influenza (to "stimulate your immune system"); vitamin C; and laetrile for "short-term response—relief from pain, remission of malignancy." (The continued use of laetrile surprises me, because the majority of alternative specialists, even the most adventuresome, agree that it has been proven ineffective.)

If you're a cancer patient, how should you expect to react to the Gerson treatment, as described above? Within three to ten days, you'll probably develop the following flu-like symptoms: fever, nausea, vomiting, stomach cramps, weakness, dizziness, cold sores, fever blisters, and headache—first every two weeks, then every month for the duration of the treatment. This misery is expected and actually welcomed by the Gerson therapists, who attribute it to an "allergic inflammation," a manifestation of the body's innate healing powers—"proof" that the therapy is working, detoxifying sick tissue, restoring vitality. Whenever it happens, treatment is stopped for a few days and then resumed. Conventional doctors think it's the result of the drastic change in diet and the effect of all the additional supplements.

My personal reaction to this entire scenario is "Thanks, but no thanks." I cannot imagine anyone, sick or well, running from the juicer to the table to the medicine chest to the toilet so many times a day. But at last count, some 600 people were doing so every year at the Gerson clinic. Whether or not this treatment prolongs life, it would certainly seem so to anyone enduring it.

If you decide to go the Gerson route, plan to remain at the clinic for three to eight weeks, depending on how you respond. The cost is about $4,000 a week for you, and several hundred more for your companion. Expect to continue treatment for about two years after you get home. Your food bills will then amount to at least $300 a week, and the supplements will cost another $200 per month. It's not cheap, but it's not nearly as expensive as hospitalization and chemotherapy.

What claims did Gerson himself make for his regimen, and what are his successors saying? How are their results assessed by the scientific community?

Although Gerson published many papers over the years, his best-known work was the book *A Cancer Therapy: Results of Fifty Cases* (Gerson Institute, 5th ed., 1986), in which he concluded that "there is an effective treatment of cancer, even in advanced cases." His last statement, published after his death in 1959, reported a "success" rate of about 50 percent for his regimen. The doctors currently running the Gerson clinic say they're seeing significant "responses" and cures in advanced cases—not only of cancer, but also of heart disease and arthritis. According to Norman Fritz, the clinic's vice president at the Gerson Institute in Bonita, California, melanoma and lung cancer can be cured in as many as 90 percent of cases even after they have spread, and patients with brain tumors have a 30 percent cure rate. The Gerson monthly, *Healing Newsletter,* publishes testimonials from patients providing details of these cures. However, other statements from the institute itself are more modest and suggest that the Gerson method works best when combined with standard anticancer treatment. That's an important departure from Gerson's original stance.

For the most part, the scientific community gives the Gerson method thumbs down. Conventional oncologists insist that his theories are erroneous, and that the side effects of his treatment are serious and unacceptable. Analysis of the fifty case reports in his book indicates that some of the "cures" in fact occurred in patients who had received conventional treatment before they ever went to Gerson; other cases had not been diagnosed by biopsy and may not have been cancer at all. However, during Senate hearings in Washington at which Gerson was invited to testify, five independent doctors stated that they were impressed with how well their patients responded to his therapy. Three British reviewers who visited the Gerson clinic in 1989 and studied the records of 149 patients concluded that many received impressive *subjective* benefits, presumably because of their commitment to the program and their determination to overcome their disease. Although there were some reports of tumor shrinkage, these reviewers found little, if any, data confirming that the Gerson regimen had a measurable, physical effect on cancer.

Does the Gerson method sound like something you'd try if your life was on the line? Are you deterred by the fact that doing it "by their book" is demanding and arduous, not to mention expensive, full of side effects, and offers results that have been dismissed by the scientific community? I don't think I personally would or could undertake such a program. But I also believe there should be additional, intensive research into some of the theories proposed by Gerson. Here's why:

- It's not enough simply to criticize Gerson's method because it's tough to follow. Also, although I agree that some of the data are flawed, there are too many testimonials for us to ignore them. I've never spoken to anyone who doubts that Gerson was honest and sincere. He was also well trained, and a keen observer. It's inconceivable to me that *all* his conclusions were flawed, and that there is no validity whatsoever to any of his claims. Further investigation should be carried out, not only by Gerson-type institutes but by the scientific community, under the leadership of the cancer branch of the National Institutes of Health. There would then be no recriminations or accusations concerning the way any of the studies were conducted, and little dispute over whether or not their conclusions were valid.

- The Gerson diet—high in carbohydrates and low in fat—is what every modern study has shown to be effective in preventing some cancers. The rationale for adding potassium and restricting sodium is also gaining theoretical credibility. Cancer of the colon is often accompanied by low potassium levels; recent experiments have shown that cells can be damaged by a lack of potassium, and that normal function is restored when adequate amounts are provided. Furthermore, the cellular content of potassium and sodium appears to influence growth and multiplication of cells.

- The enzymes and potassium-rich minerals in those hourly juice drinks (together with the pressed calves' liver that was originally included) are great sources of vitamin A, believed to have anticancer properties. Also, the iron and copper in these nutrients may stimulate function of the T cells and other cellular constituents of the immune system that play a role in controlling cancer.

- The coffee enema in the regimen draws the most ridicule from Gerson's critics (see chapter 18). But Gerson emphasized its importance at a time when mainstream surgeons were giving their patients coffee enemas to treat shock and postoperative bleeding. So, as originally conceived, the coffee enema was by no means "off the wall." Also, coffee enemas may increase the absorption of vitamin A, in which the Gerson diet is rich. This, in turn, may enhance the efficiency of the immune system by stimulating protective "killer cells" to destroy cancerous tissue. Furthermore, patients insist that these coffee enemas do lessen pain and thus reduce the need for painkilling drugs, which can harm the liver.

- Investigators have shown that supplemental thyroid increases resistance to infection, and that added iodine neutralizes the action of hormones that may promote the unbridled growth of cancer cells.
- A diet rich in potassium and low in sodium increases aldosterone, a steroid hormone that retards the growth of some tumors.

So you see that what starts off as a seemingly ridiculous approach may have an acceptable theoretical rationale. That's why it's so important to evaluate the Gerson diet properly and not dismiss it out of hand.

❖ ❖ ❖   What's the bottom line with respect to the Gerson method? At the moment, I believe that it is too trying and taxing for most people, especially those with cancer. If you decide to go to the clinic in Tijuana, do not abandon other forms of therapy that your doctor believes may help slow down the progress of your disease. Some of the dietary prescriptions recommended by Gerson, such as the emphasis on carbohydrates and the reduction of fat and protein, make sense. Coffee enemas, on the other hand, are not my cup of tea! Most important, we must encourage the establishment to test Gerson's theories. The stakes are too high to ignore them.

The rigorous, demanding Gerson program sits well with some who try it because it gives them hope—regardless of the outcome. The reaction of one man, the father of a young woman who had breast cancer that had spread widely, reflects the attitude (and the dilemma) of such patients and their families. After all the conventional treatments had failed, he took his daughter to the Gerson clinic. She entered the program determined to make it work, for this was her last chance. She received no promises of cure, but she was given hope—and remained convinced throughout her stay that she would be healed. The outcome is irrelevant. What's important is that her remaining months and years were free of despair. How many conventional regimens do as much for their patients?

Megadose Vitamin C

The mainstream medical community says that there is no scientific proof that huge doses of vitamin C can help treat and prevent the common cold. So why do so many doctors, including me, not only take it themselves but give it to their family and friends (though not their patients)? Because there's always the chance that the "establishment" is wrong! There is an equally heated controversy about the usefulness of megadoses of vitamin C in the treatment of cancer, and here, as in the case of the common cold, I am told that there is also significant surreptitious use of this vitamin.

The late Linus Pauling, and now his associates, are at the center of the dispute over vitamin C. Although there was speculation in the medical community for many years that vitamin C might have a favorable impact on cancer, it was the book *Cancer and Vitamin C,* written in 1979 by Linus Pauling and Ewan Cameron, that brought this possibility to the public's attention. Pauling and his associates recommend more than 200 times the official minimum daily requirement of 45 milligrams of vitamin C—a minimum of 10,000 milligrams daily for cancer patients. The initial dose is 1,000 to 2,000 milligrams a day; this is gradually increased to the goal of 10,000 milligrams. Should the patient develop diarrhea (the most common side effect of megadose vitamin C), the dosage is cut back.

Pauling and Cameron presented statistics purporting to show that megadoses of vitamin C are beneficial in treating virtually every kind of cancer, as a result of two major mechanisms. First, they claimed that it inhibits the formation of hyaluronidase, an enzyme that facilitates the spread of cancer. It also increases the production of collagen, normal connective tissue that cancer cells must penetrate in order to spread, or metastasize. The more collagen there is, the less easily and the less quickly these cells can spread.

Establishment scientists do not agree with Pauling's theories, statistics, or conclusions. In view of Pauling's sterling credentials, researchers at the Mayo Clinic undertook an impressive study to test his hypothesis about vitamin C. They concluded that it had no effect in the cancer patients they treated. Pauling retorted that the Mayo study was invalid because the patients selected had all previously received immunosuppressive therapy, which compromised their ability to react favorably to vitamin C. Fair enough. So the Mayo researchers launched a second investigation. Again, their findings did not substantiate those of Pauling, who once more objected. This time he claimed that after the Mayo Clinic researchers had decided that the vitamin C wasn't working, they stopped it abruptly, and in so doing reduced patients' resistance to infection and enhanced the spread of their cancer. Pauling and Cameron had one other objection. They felt very strongly that their hypothesis should be tested at more than one center. So a third trial was conducted, at several cancer centers. This time, the researchers found that large doses of vitamin C may improve patients' sense of well-being but do not prolong their survival.

Proponents of vitamin C continue to claim that it slows down the progress of cancer but does not cure it. They say that patients who take vitamin C in the high doses they recommend are better able to tolerate conventional chemotherapy and radiation, and that they live longer and in greater comfort.

Most doctors used to think that megadoses of vitamin C were harmless, and at worst only a waste of money. However, it now appears that if you have a personal or family history of kidney stones, too much vitamin C may contribute to their formation. That's because an intake of more than 1,000 milligrams per day can cause a buildup of calcium oxalate in the urine, the most common constituent of kidney stones. Megadoses of vitamin C can also damage various body tissues by causing abnormal amounts of iron to be deposited in them and can also cause too much urate in the urine, which can result in stone formation.

Recently, researchers at the National Institute of Diabetes and Digestive and Kidney Diseases of the NIH have decided, on the basis of a federally sponsored study, that for healthy people, the optimal daily intake of vitamin C is 200 milligrams, not the current RDA of 45 milligrams, but that doses greater than 400 milligrams "have no evident value." They issued no statement about the use of vitamin C in the management of cancer.

❖ ❖ ❖   That's the vitamin C story to date. What's the bottom line? The most recent research indicates that megadose vitamin C does nothing for patients with advanced cancer, and that doses in excess of 1,000 milligrams a day are not only wasted, but may cause diarrhea, stomach trouble, kidney stones, and iron overload.

Several other cancer therapies, all of which are controversial, incorporate dietary regimens. Some have for the most part been abandoned, even by the alternative medicine community. Others continue to be used and have passionate followers. In the opinion of mainstream medicine, none has been shown to have any anticancer effect. Despite all the hype, advanced cancers of the lung, pancreas, colon, or prostate have not been shown to be cured by any of the following, but some of them are described for their historic interest.

The Hoxsey Treatment

In the 1840s, an American farmer named John Hoxsey observed that some of his horses that had developed tumors were cured after grazing on certain grasses and wild plants. He made mixtures of these plants, added some herbal home remedies, and supplied the final mélange to other farmers whose horses were ailing. John Hoxsey bequeathed this formula to his son, who passed it along to his descendants. One of them, a veterinary surgeon, used it routinely in his practice. Before he died, he suggested to his son, Harry Hoxsey, that he try it on humans with cancer. Harry Hoxsey opened the first Hoxsey cancer clinic in Dallas. Its fame spread, and between 1920 and 1950, many other such centers were established in seventeen states. At one point, 10,000 patients were taking the Hoxsey therapy, whose complete formula, incidentally, has never been disclosed. After investigation by the FDA and criticism from the scientific community, all the Hoxsey clinics in the United States were closed in the late 1950s. However, I understand that Hoxsey's onetime nurse continues to run a clinic in Tijuana, Mexico.

Hoxsey offered some dietary advice along with his potion: no pork, tomatoes, pickles (or any food with vinegar), salt, sugar, artificial sweeteners, alcohol, bleached flour, or carbonated beverages. In addition to an "herbal tonic" or paste, all of Hoxsey's patients were treated for fungus (*Candida*), and given a variety of vitamins, calcium supplements, laxatives, and antiseptic douches. If you go to the current Tijuana clinic looking for a cancer cure, you'll stay for about three days, with a follow-up visit in three to six months.

As far as I can determine, Harry Hoxsey never attempted to offer any scientific rationale for his treatment and never claimed that he understood the causes of cancer. He did, however, theorize that cancer was due to a "chemical imbalance" in the body, which, he believed, made newborn cells cancerous. He thought that normalizing the body fluids with his herbal preparations and the dietary changes he recommended could cure cancers that had not yet spread.

You've probably concluded that I think all this Hoxsey stuff is hogwash. Well, I did, until I started reviewing the literature on the subject. To my surprise, I found that respected scientific researchers suspect that he may have been on to something! For example, Frederick Mohs, the originator of the widely used Mohs's chemosurgical technique, found that certain ingredients in Hoxsey's paste cured nonmelanoma skin cancers. He also determined that they are effective in 99 percent of basal cell cancers. Although Mohs later excised these cancers by means of a special surgical technique, there is no escaping the fact that the ingredients in Hoxsey's paste—notably zinc chloride, antimony trisulfide, and bloodroot (*Sanguinaria canadensis,* used by American Indians to treat nasal polyps, warts, and cancer)—have some effect. What about the tonic and preparations taken internally for other kinds of cancers? After evaluating (in animals) many of the herbs (they contain burdock, buckthorn, cascara, barberry, licorice, red clover, pokeroot, prickly ash, stillingia), the National Cancer Institute concluded that some do have antitumor properties. So it's possible that using these herbs together yields more impressive results than giving any of them alone. None of them has side effects in humans when taken in the doses recommended by Hoxsey, though overdosing can cause poisoning. Their anticancer potential for humans requires further study.

Therapists at the Hoxsey clinic claim they can cure 80 percent of their patients who have the proper "attitude." There have been no formal clinical trials at the clinic, but visiting doctors who have reviewed its patients' charts have come up with mixed results. One such group concluded that the Hoxsey method "successfully treats pathologically-proven cases of cancer, both internal and external, without the use of surgery, radium, or X-ray, and is superior to such conventional methods." However, another committee, this one composed of doctors from the University of British Columbia, who studied the records of seventy-eight patients treated at the Hoxsey clinic, reached a totally different conclusion. They found that in more than half the cases, either the cancer progressed or the patient died; in one quarter of the group, the diagnosis of cancer had never really been established; one-tenth had received prior treatment that could conceivably have cured their cancer before they ever reached the Hoxsey clinic; and only one patient was cured—of a skin cancer that can be cured by any one of several conventional approaches.

Over the years there have been charges and counter-charges, by the National Cancer Institute and the AMA on the one hand and advocates of the Hoxsey treatment on the other, each accusing the other of bad faith and worse.

❖ ❖ ❖ The bottom line on the Hoxsey treatment? It seems to me that there is enough evidence to warrant an independent, careful evaluation of the Hoxsey method, even though I am personally not impressed with the data and results to date. What should you do in the meantime? Do not abandon other therapies, even alternative therapies, for the Hoxsey method.

The Livingstone-Wheeler Treatment

Virginia Livingstone-Wheeler, who died in 1990, was a distinguished establishment physician and scientist who developed a theory of the causation of cancer based on personal observations made in her laboratory. Her work has been carefully assessed by the academic community.

Livingstone, a graduate of the New York University Medical School, later became associate professor in the Bureau of Biological Research at Rutgers University and held senior academic posts elsewhere as well. While studying cancerous tissue under the microscope, she detected microorganisms of different shapes and sizes. After evaluating them for years, she decided that they were varying forms of the same bacterium and named it *P. cryptocides*. Even though this bacterium was occasionally present, in small numbers, in healthy tissue, Livingstone concluded that it plays a role in the development of cancer. She postulated that when the body's resistance is lowered, for whatever reason, this organism multiplies and eventually overwhelms the patient's defense mechanisms. To prove her point, she inoculated various animals with *P. cryptocides* and claimed that it did indeed cause cancer. Her book *The Conquest of Cancer* explains her theory in detail.

The logical next step for Livingstone, given her conviction that *P. cryptocides* causes cancer, was to develop a vaccine against it. She did so, and established a clinic where she vaccinated cancer patients. The results were controversial.

In addition to the vaccine, the Livingstone regimen—like almost every other alternative anticancer diet—emphasizes whole grains, fresh vegetables, and fruit. Smoked meat and poultry, alcohol, coffee, refined sugars, and processed foods are all banned. Megadose vitamins, minerals, and digestive enzymes are also prescribed, as are daily coffee enemas for "detoxification."

Since Livingstone's death in 1990, her work has been continued at the Livingstone Clinic in California. I am told it is popular and well attended. The basic treatment consists of a series of vaccines to boost immunity, transfusions of whole blood from family members and friends, and other substances used in conventional cancer centers: interferon, tumor necrosis factor, thymosin, gamma globulin, and agents that act on the immune system. Its thrust, however, remains the conquest of the tiny organism whose role in cancer Livingstone dedicated her professional life to investigating.

Most of Livingstone's peers do not agree with her interpretation of what she saw under the microscope. They believe that *P. cryptocides* is not a new organism but merely variant strains of staphylococcus and streptococcus, both commonly present in many body tissues, healthy and diseased. However, one of Livingstone's findings *has* been confirmed by others. When her microorganisms are grown in a test tube, they produce a hormone similar to one found in healthy humans as well as in people with certain cancers. It is possible that an antibiotic, or some other substance that eradicates *P. cryptocides,* suppresses the formation of this hormone, thus slowing down or preventing the growth of cancer. This is all quite theoretical, but it indicates, once more, that we are just beginning to scratch the surface in our understanding of the many different ways cancer can begin, grow, and kill, and how important it is to follow every research lead. Simply scoffing at a theory, ignoring it, or calling the people who propose it quacks and fakes is not the way to go about conquering cancer.

❖ ❖ ❖   What's the bottom line on the Livingstone treatment? There's no harm, in my view, in accepting it if it doesn't deter you from proven, effective treatment (of which there is precious little against most advanced cancers). However, the vaccines it employs can, at least theoretically, cause allergic reactions. Blood transfusions, too, are not without risk, even when the blood is donated by your own grandmother. And here's an interesting twist. A few years ago, some researchers compared the outcomes of a large number of patients with far-advanced cancer: some treated at a large conventional university hospital, and others at the Livingstone Clinic. They found no difference in survival between the two groups. However, the quality of life was better—guess where? At the university hospital. This is one of the few instances where alternative medicine lost out in that respect.

The Kelley (Gonzalez) Regimen

To end this chapter, here's an example of another "offbeat" nutritional treatment for cancer. In the 1970s, the Kelley regimen was one of the best-known and most popular unconventional dietary treatments for cancer. It had originated in the early 1960s, when William Kelley, an orthodontist, was told by his doctor that he had pancreatic cancer, a malignancy that is invariably fatal within five years. Preoccupied with his illness, he began to speculate why people develop cancer. After reviewing all the available literature, he concluded that it was because of some derangement in the way the body handles protein. Enzymes that digest protein are produced in the pancreas, from which they either enter the intestine to help digest food, or are secreted directly into the bloodstream. This latter route bypasses the gut and delivers the enzymes to all the cells of the body, whose proteins they mistakenly digest. Kelley devised a test purporting to evaluate the body's protein status, and so to detect the presence of cancer and determine how long it has been there. He also claimed that his test could determine whether a subject is *vulnerable* to malignancy, in which event cancer might be prevented. Kelley decided that he'd had his own tumor for a long time, even though, as best I can make out from the literature, his diagnosis was never confirmed. On the basis of the results of his diagnostic test, Kelley concluded that his wife and two of his children also had cancer. (Now there's self-confidence for you!) He treated himself and the other "stricken" members of his family, and they all lived happily ever after. What a saga!

Kelley believed that the wrong diet and environmental pollutants cause derangement of protein metabolism. He devised a corrective diet that was quite variable, depending on where you fell on his scale of vulnerability. Some persons were advised to follow a purely vegetarian diet, while others were prescribed lots of red meat. He established a booming mail-order business, from which one could buy the test material for self-diagnosis and the enzymes needed to digest protein properly.

The Kelley regimen is no longer being practiced as such. Despite the many claims he made for it while he was in business, he stated in the 1980s, shortly before he retired, that he had never meant for it to be used to treat cancer; that he was not a physician but a dentist, and that he was merely making dietary and nutritional recommendations he hoped would enhance health.

Kelley's work has since been analyzed by Nicolas Gonzalez, a New York physician trained in immunology. Gonzalez believes that several aspects of the Kelley regimen make sense, especially the nutritional recommendations. Gonzalez places great importance on individual variability, and unlike Gerson or Livingstone, he believes that every patient requires his or her own personal dietary prescription. However, like Kelley, he pushes supplements such as hydrochloric acid and protein-digesting enzymes, raw beef organs and glands, and the same vigorous detoxification with coffee enemas that is the hallmark of virtually every alternative cancer treatment.

Gonzalez was drawn to Kelley's hypothesis after carefully studying the records of fifty of Kelley's patients. That task took the better part of five years to complete, and Gonzalez reported his results in a 500-page volume. He was apparently encouraged by the fact that several of Kelley's cancer patients had survived for ten years or more. He also found that twenty-two of his own patients with pancreatic cancer who followed the prescribed regimen lived an average of nine years. (Among conventionally treated patients with pancreatic cancer, there are few survivors after five years; in fact, most patients die within twelve months.)

The records of Kelley's fifty patients, which had so impressed Gonzalez, were submitted for review to six other doctors, of whom three were mainstream types and the other three "alternatives." Their analyses followed party lines. The mainstream doctors were, for the most part, unimpressed. They thought the results could be explained by the benefits of previous conventional therapy, or that the results fell within the accepted variability in behavior that some cancers show anyway. The unconventional analysts were more enthusiastic.

❖ ❖ ❖ The bottom line? I'm withholding judgment. I understand that the National Cancer Institute is currently looking into Gonzalez's work, and I look forward to learning their results.

As you read the descriptions of the various dietary alternatives to the treatment of cancer and compare their results with those obtained by mainstream approaches, remember that the track record of conventional approaches is not very impressive. No practitioners can rest on their laurels. Doctors who ridicule complementary regimens do not, in most cases, have anything better to offer.

There is no doubt that some alternative regimens seem to improve the quality of life, but none seems to prolong it. Perhaps quality of life is better because patients feel they have greater control of their lives. In many cases, they're treated in a more caring, attentive, hands-on way, and maybe that makes a difference too. They attend classes, seminars, follow-up evaluations, and other kinds of support sessions. The very intensity of it all can be therapeutic. Contrast all of this with the conventional treatment of cancer, in which the patient is given a pill, or an injection, or an X-ray beam, often from a technician, without receiving any reassurance or comfort from the doctor, and is then sent home to ruminate, to suffer, and to die. Active participation in your therapy—even if it's detoxification, whose effectiveness is moot; or squeezing raw juices; or taking a hundred pills a day—keeps you busy and full of hope. Who can be sure that this attitude in itself doesn't have a positive effect against cancer?

❖ 15 ❖

ENZYMES

Is Enough Really Enough?

Conventional doctors give you enzyme supplements only when you are deficient in them. However, many alternative practitioners recommend the routine, universal consumption of enzymes to "improve digestion," and to prevent or alleviate a wide variety of diseases. The shelves of health food stores are bursting with these products—Nature's Plus Digestive Enzymes, Solgar's Vegetarian Digestive Aid, Megafood Super Potency Digestive Enzymes, Twinlabs SuperEnzyme Caps, Schiff Enzyme, and many others. Is there any proof that enzyme supplements do anything for you? Is there a downside to taking extra enzymes when your body is presumably making enough?

Enzymes are proteins that act as catalysts for virtually all biological and chemical reactions in the body, of which the digestive process is one of the most important. Enzymes do not initiate these reactions, but they accelerate the rate at which they occur. Many critical biological interactions would not proceed without them. The enzymes themselves require certain nutrient helpers, called coenzymes—such as vitamins, minerals, and other proteins—before they can perform their functions. Once an enzyme has participated in a given reaction (for example, a digestive process), it must be replenished. Every cell in the body contains some 100,000 enzymes, of which many must be derived from food.

Enzymes break down every component of the food we eat—proteins, fats, and carbohydrates—and are produced in various parts of the body. Enzymes in the mouth are made by salivary glands; in the stomach by specialized cells; but the most important enzymes come from the pancreas. If the pancreas is chronically infected or has been damaged by disease or a congenital disorder, it may not be able to make enough of these critical enzymes. When that happens, much of the fat, protein, and carbohydrate you eat remains undigested and simply passes through the gut and out of the body without having been absorbed. The result is a nutritional zero. To prevent such malabsorption, physicians prescribe enzyme replacement therapy. A classic example is the treatment of cystic fibrosis, in which the ducts that carry the enzymes from the pancreas are plugged by abnormal secretions. The pancreatic fluid containing the enzymes, unable to leave the pancreas, backs up into it and eventually destroys large areas within it where the enzyme is made. So not only are the enzymes held back by these blocked ducts, but their production is also eventually decreased. The resulting enzyme deficiency leads to malabsorption, diarrhea, and malnutrition. In such cases, replacement therapy is lifesaving.

Other digestive enzymes are produced farther down in the intestinal tract, and act at different sites than those from the pancreas. For example, there is lactase, which breaks down lactose (the sugar present in milk and milk products). When there's not enough lactase around, the lactose you eat is not absorbed. It moves down the intestinal tract intact, producing abnormal amounts of gas, bloating, cramping, and diarrhea. Most people throughout the world (with the notable exception of Scandinavians) have some degree of lactase deficiency and are therefore lactose-intolerant. However, this is not a life-threatening situation, and the treatment is very simple. You can replace lactase with over-the-counter tablets from a pharmacy or health food store, and lactose-supplemented dairy products are available at grocery stores.

Alpha galactodase is another common, though less well known, enzyme whose deficiency plagues many of us. The symptoms are, again, a surfeit of gas, cramping, diarrhea, and other intestinal complaints. These are most likely to occur after eating beans, legumes, and cruciferous vegetables such as cauliflower and cabbage. Like lactase, alpha galactodase is commercially available without a prescription, as a product called Beano. But don't take it without your doctor's okay, because Beano is produced from mold and may make you sick if you happen to be allergic to penicillin. It can also interfere with sugar metabolism, so check with your doctor if you're diabetic.

There is no controversy about replacing any enzyme when it's lacking. However, conventional physicians and alternative practitioners part company when the latter prescribe "pancreatic enzyme therapy" for a wide variety of "conditions" in which these enzymes are not lacking. Because enzymes normally break down so many different kinds of molecules, proponents of universal supplementation hold that they should also be used to attack cancers, areas of inflammation, infectious agents, and abnormal tissues. They believe that enzymes dissolve the coating of cancer cells, allowing white blood corpuscles and other components of the immune system, or even anticancer drugs, to invade and destroy them. This particular concept is particularly popular in Germany. Pancreatic enzymes are also claimed to kill several different kinds of viruses, including those that cause AIDS, by digesting their protein coat and ostensibly leaving them at the mercy of the body's natural defenses. So "believing" practitioners administer pancreatic enzymes, either by mouth or by injection, to persons with such diverse conditions as cancer, multiple sclerosis, arthritis, viral infections, athletic injuries, and—most recently—AIDS.

There's more. These enthusiasts say that enzymes are good for you even if you are perfectly healthy and are not deficient in them. They recommend plant-derived supplements similar to those our bodies produce—protease, amylase, and lactase—as well as cellulase, an enzyme unique to plants that digests fiber. The enthusiasts reason we can derive nutritional benefits from the fiber broken down by cellulase. Personally, I'd rather have my fiber intact, so that it can exert its many beneficial actions as it moves through the colon. The pro-enzyme folks also claim that eating more enzymes leaves your healthy, normally functioning pancreas with less work to do.

There is another mechanism by which plant enzymes are thought to help the pancreas. Digestion begins in the stomach, where hydrochloric acid and a weaker digestive enzyme called gastrin act on what you've eaten. Pancreatic enzymes do not take part in this process, because they are not present in the stomach. However, plant enzymes in fruit and raw vegetables, nuts, and seeds (or in their supplements) act on food while it's still in the stomach and help predigest it. As a result of this predigestion, by the time the food gets into the duodenum (the first part of the small intestine), ready to be digested by the pancreatic enzymes waiting there, some of it has already been broken down. Consequently, the pancreas has fewer enzymes to make. A pancreas with less work to do has more time to rest, and accordingly is a happier, healthier pancreas—or so the theory goes.

All this sounds plausible on the surface. But there are two flaws to these conclusions: (1) none of this speculation has ever been proven; and (2) most plant enzymes are deactivated by the stomach acid the moment they arrive in the stomach and so don't really do any predigesting. In response to these objections, "enzymologists" insist that there isn't enough acid in the stomach to neutralize all the plant enzymes for the first hour after food is ingested. During that interval, they say that the enzymes can digest 30 to 40 percent of the starches, 30 percent of the protein, and 10 percent of the fat. If you consume only cooked food, and no plant supplements, you lose the benefit of this predigestion, and the consequences can be pretty awful, they say. (Pasteurization, canning, microwaving, and cooking to temperatures above 118 degrees Fahrenheit deactivate these plant enzymes.) Since your pancreas must now make more enzymes, it becomes enlarged, functions less efficiently, and is eventually unable to maintain production. As a consequence, your digestion is impaired and your colon becomes "toxic" and laden with poisonous wastes that eventually make their way to the liver. Your liver, too, then becomes "sick." All of this leads to the breakdown of the immune system, leaving the body vulnerable to such diverse disorders as infection, cancer, allergies, sciatica, and acne—you name it. All that just from eating cooked food and no enzymes!

I don't buy any of this domino theory. I have never heard of a pancreas becoming "hypertrophied" (enlarged) from overuse. The pancreas is not a muscle. Some of its component cells can be damaged by autoimmune disorders, infections, or cancer, but there is no scientific evidence that the pancreas becomes enlarged and fails to function properly because you don't eat enough raw fruit and vegetables or because you cook your food. There are millions and millions of people who do just that and have perfectly normal pancreases. Mind you, I heartily endorse liberal consumption of fresh fruit and vegetables, but supplements are another matter, especially if you already eat at least five, and preferably seven, servings per day of the natural food.

❖ ❖ ❖ What's the bottom line? If you have a digestive problem due to some disease of the pancreas, or cystic fibrosis, or lactose intolerance, enzyme replacement is a must. Raw fruits and vegetables are the staff of life; they're nutritious—chock-full of antioxidants, minerals, vitamins, fiber, and other phytochemicals. If you can't get enough of them in your diet, enzyme supplements can be beneficial—but not otherwise. And don't expect any supplemental enzymes, no matter how you take them, to cure infections, arthritis, cancer, or anything else.

❖ 16 ❖

FASTING

Even When You're Thin?

What did both Moses and Jesus do that the Koran also endorses "so that you may safeguard yourselves against every kind of ill and become righteous"? They fasted—deliberately abstained from food—a practice that has persisted over the millennia in many different cultures and civilizations.

The definitions of a "fast" and its duration vary, depending on why it is being done and by whom it has been prescribed. If it isn't because of Lent, Yom Kippur, or Ramadan, or a hunger strike to protest something or other, people these days fast to lose weight, to prove to themselves that they have self-discipline, to "detoxify" the body, or to "rest" the digestive tract. Many people fast simply because they believe that it's a good thing to do "now and then." Mainstream doctors rarely prescribe fasting. They spend more time answering questions from religious patients who want to know if it's safe to fast on a particular religious occasion, or to skip a certain medication on that day. However, although there are few if any documented physiological reasons for fasting, it is nevertheless commonly recommended by many holistic practitioners. What's more, there are clinics and spas throughout the world where you pay a fortune to go hungry.

Does fasting do any good? Occasionally, when a food allergy is suspected of causing an unexplained symptom—such as chronic headache—fasting, followed by the reintroduction of various foods, one at a time, can help identify the culprit substance. Russian doctors have claimed a 70 percent success rate treating schizophrenic patients by withholding all food for about a month. During this time, the patients quell their hunger by drinking at least a quart of water every day. Although fasting does not cure their schizophrenia, the patients are calmer, and their behavior is less bizarre. These observations were confirmed in a study at a psychiatric hospital in New York City. However, fasting is not widely used in the treatment of schizophrenia in this country because remission is neither prolonged nor its duration predictable, and similar or better results are obtained with psychopharmacology. But I am nevertheless fascinated that fasting has any impact at all on this psychiatric disorder, and I cannot explain it. It is possible that fasting leads to changes in body chemistry that modify one or more of the mechanisms contributing to schizophrenia. It may also be that fasting eliminates an undetected food allergy. There have also been scattered accounts, most of them anecdotal, that periodic fasting alleviates the symptoms of rheumatoid arthritis. Some of my patients have told me that their joint pains do ease up temporarily after they fast for a day or two. Perhaps during that time, they too are avoiding some substance to which they are allergic.

Some claims for fasting are ridiculous: for example, the claim that it can cure gonorrhea, or that it produces a hormone that stimulates the immune system. No such hormone has ever been identified, and the only thing that will cure gonorrhea is the appropriate antibiotic.

What theories are offered to explain the claimed benefits of fasting? According to one theory, fasting "rests" the intestinal tract. I was raised in the old school of "use it or lose it." Doctors prescribe exercise—not rest—for health and well-being. Regular physical activity is good for the heart, lungs, legs, muscles, and other parts of the body, not to mention the libido. Still, as far as the intestinal tract is concerned, a short fast may be desirable when the gut is inflamed (if you've got, say, gastritis or diverticulitis) or has been hit by a twenty-four-hour bug. But don't try fasting if you have an acute ulcer, because food buffers stomach acid. This acid accumulates in an empty stomach, and it will have you climbing the walls with pain.

Another theory has it that when you don't eat, the energy your body would normally expend on digestion can be devoted to "healing" whatever ails you. Far-fetched!

There are various fasting regimens, all of which permit fluids—plain or distilled water, herbal teas, or juices (see chapter 23). Naturopaths (holistic practitioners who employ natural methods and diets to prevent and treat disease: they are N.D.s, not M.D.s) most often recommend the vegetable juice fast (to which small amounts of fruit juice are added). This fast is the one used at the popular Birchner-Benner clinic in Zurich. It's also the safest way to fast, because these juices are loaded with vitamins, minerals, amino acids, natural sugars, and food enzymes, all of which can be utilized by the body, especially important when other nutrients are unavailable. However, some naturopaths strenuously oppose it because they view juice as food, which, in their view, defeats the purpose of the fast. Instead of vegetable juice, they prescribe enough water—plain, distilled, or from a spring—to control thirst, insisting on a minimum of three eight-ounce glasses a day. Once the fast is over, they reintroduce food very gradually. These practitioners generally recommend two such fasts a year, each lasting five days.

Here, *according to naturopaths,* are the biological changes that occur when you're fasting:

- You consume fewer "toxins," and your body continues to eliminate those that are already present. This leaves you as clean and pure as the driven snow.
- Since you're eating no fats, the viscosity of your blood is reduced. Thinner blood delivers nutrients more efficiently to the body tissues.
- You divert energy from your dormant digestive process toward strengthening your immune system.

That's what the naturopaths say. Let me tell you what I believe *really* happens when you're fasting:

- Your blood sugar level drops. In order to obtain enough energy to function, your body utilizes protein, of which muscle is a very rich source. The longer the fast, the more muscle is broken down, and the more ammonia and nitrogen, the end products of its breakdown, are produced. Their higher concentration in your blood, brain, and other tissues leaves you feeling really lousy—nauseated, weak, tired, and depressed. (Proponents of fasting say these symptoms prove that "toxins"—never identified—are leaving the body.) Normally, your kidneys and liver can eliminate excess ammonia or nitrogen from your body. But when you're fasting, these organs too are undernourished and work less efficiently. So the real consequence of prolonged fasting is that your body actually accumulates harmful substances rather than eliminating them.

- The uric acid in your blood rises; this can bring on attacks of acute gout.
- The levels of calcium, potassium, and other minerals in your blood fall; this can affect your cardiac rhythm. You may remember hearing about several people, mostly young women, who died suddenly from the abrupt onset of a chaotic heart rhythm while following very-low-calorie diets to lose weight. Some naturopaths tell their patients to expect disturbances in their heart rhythm while fasting, and sometimes falsely reassure them that such disturbances are harmless.
- Your kidneys or liver can fail during a prolonged fast, causing death.
- You can become anemic; this leaves you *more* vulnerable to infection.
- Stopping medication during a fast can be dangerous, and even maintaining the same dose can be harmful. That's why your doctor must know if you're planning to fast, and for how long you intend to do so. The dosage requirement of medication, whether it's insulin or a heart drug, may change when you're fasting. You may need less, or occasionally more.
- Chances are that you will develop a headache while you're fasting, especially if you're prone to headaches in the first place. That's what was found in a survey of Israeli hospital employees who fasted for twenty-four hours in observance of Yom Kippur. Only 7 percent of the control group, who chose not to fast, had a headache that day; however, 39 percent of those who fasted (none of whom had a history of chronic headache) developed one.

◆ ◆ ◆

There are real hazards associated with prolonged fasting. It doesn't surprise me that at one "fasting clinic," where patients were given only distilled water for thirty days in order to "purify" the body, at least six people died over a five-year period. (The courts held the therapists responsible for these deaths.) So don't rush to join the fasting band-wagon, especially if you have any problem with your heart, kidneys, or lungs, or if you are pregnant, nursing, or dia-betic. And don't force anyone in your family, especially a child, to fast. Remember that—unlike some other forms of alternative medicine, which can do no harm—fasting can be hazardous.

❖ ❖ ❖   What's the bottom line about fasting?

• If you're a devout Jew or Muslim and want to fast on your religious holidays, discuss it with your doctor, especially if you have some health problem or are taking any medica-tion.
• If you've been on a drinking or eating binge and want to reset your "appestat," fasting for a day or two may make you feel better. But don't fast to cure obesity. That requires more than periodic self-denial. You need a lifelong plan of sensible eating; you can't fast forever.

❖ 17 ❖

HERBAL THERAPY
Dedicated to My Son Herb

Before the era of modern pharmaceutics, doctors used to treat their patients with plants, particularly herbs. That's all they had, and they did a credible job with them, all things considered. In those days, there was no FDA, and there was no requirement for double-blind trials before a medicine could be used. Anecdotal accounts of the benefits of a botanical agent, handed down from generation to generation, constituted all the evidence doctors had—or needed—before using it to heal the sick. For example, in the seventeenth century, natives in the jungles of Peru told a Jesuit priest living among them that the bark of a local tree could lower fever. They showed him a few cases, he was convinced, and he tried it on some feverish, sick people. It worked. That observation changed the course of history and human suffering, because the active ingredient in the bark was quinine, which is still used to treat malaria, the most common disease of man.

Today, only one of every 140 mainstream physicians in this country views herbal medicine seriously. But even though your own doctor may never have prescribed herbs for you, statistics suggest that you or someone in your family is probably taking one or more of them. So, probably, is your doctor!

Although you can buy herbs as fresh leaves and roots, most people get them in the form of tablets, powders, drinks, or capsules. You can take them internally, apply them as compresses or lotions, or inhale their vapors.

They may not bear a fancy medical pedigree, but plants, roots, herbs, and flowers play an important role in the prevention and treatment of disease. Although the term "botanicals" brings to mind colorful boxes and packages on the shelves of a health food store, botanicals are the source of many drugs prescribed and being developed today. Here are a few examples:

- Digoxin, the most widely prescribed heart medication (from foxglove)
- Vincristine and vinblastine, potent anticancer drugs (from the periwinkle plant)
- Morphine, codeine, and related painkillers (from the opium poppy)
- Atropine, an important antispasmodic and cardiac drug (from belladonna)
- Penicillin, the first antibiotic (from mold)
- Aspirin—of which you take two and call your doctor in the morning (from salicin in willow bark)
- Ephedrine, the ancestor of modern antiasthma drugs (from the ephedra plant)
- Senna, the ingredient in commonly used laxatives (from the senna plant)
- Caffeine—who can start the day without it? (from the coffee bean)
- Taxol—a powerful anticancer drug (from the yew tree)

The drugs listed above are just the tip of the iceberg. So don't let the term "herbal remedy" conjure up images only of health food stores, folklore, quacks, and your great-grandparents. Herbs are the stuff of lifesaving therapy. Today, 120 commonly prescribed pharmaceuticals are extracted from 90 species of plants. Many other natural agents have been "copied" or synthesized. Hundreds of others are being used by shamans, medicine men and women, and other "nonscientific healers." To their credit, almost half the world's pharmaceutical companies are now working with "locals" on every continent, analyzing the constituents of plants heretofore ignored by the medical establishment. Now and then, one of them reaches the West and is formally approved for use. But this is a slow process. Who knows how many potentially lifesaving agents lie buried in forests and jungles around the world? And how many will never see the light of day because they are becoming extinct as our forests are replaced by "civilization"?

Notwithstanding our own "official," limited view of botanicals, 80 percent of the world still continues to depend on "primitive" herbal medicines. For these people, it's a matter of economics. They don't have the money to buy modern drugs or to support pharmaceutical research in their own countries. Despite the "nonstatus" of herbs in the eyes of mainstream medicine in this country, Americans spend well over $1 billion a year on 600 different "natural" health products (excluding teas and homeopathic medications)—a figure that is growing by 10 to 15 percent a year. Are they doing the right thing? Just because digoxin, quinine, and so many other herbal remedies are effective, does that necessarily mean that all of the hundreds now being consumed are also good? What about those that have never been tested? Are any of them potentially hazardous? Under what circumstances should you use scientifically untested herbs? Can any of them ever replace drugs prescribed by your doctor? These are some of the questions addressed in this chapter.

The *good news* about botanicals is that some have been shown to be useful, and they're usually less expensive than pharmaceuticals. Examples of some approved (or at least tolerated) by the traditional medical community include ginger (to prevent motion sickness), garlic (to lower cholesterol and blood pressure), chamomile (to promote sleep and improve digestion), and valerian (a mild sedative).

The *bad news* about herbal medicinal products is that their production remains unregulated, and there are concerns about their purity and safety. Manufacturers and importers of herbal preparations are not obliged to provide explicit information about the content and possible side effects of their products. Take ginseng, for example. The ads promise that it will improve your sex life and raise your energy level. Not only do the manufacturers fail to offer any evidence in support of these claims, they make no mention of its potential for causing insomnia, skin rashes, diarrhea, and vaginal bleeding. Other "energy boosting" herbs contain ma huang, recommended for weight reduction and to "stimulate metabolism." But check the box; you won't be told that ma huang is the Chinese name for ephedrine, a drug that can raise blood pressure, give you an irregular heartbeat, and make you nervous and jumpy. Ma huang (it's sold under various brand names, so look carefully at the label of any herbal product peddling weight loss and increased energy) has been banned in several states and has been implicated in some deaths, but it continues to be sold in most of the country without any "truth in advertising" restrictions. You'll also find kola nut and guarana in many herbal mixtures. They "stimulate" you by virtue of their caffeine content—again, something that's not usually disclosed on the label.

The vast majority of the 600 botanicals currently being sold in this country have not been scientifically tested. Their touted benefits are, for the most part, based on hearsay and testimonials. For example, while browsing in a health food store the other day, I came across a preparation called oscilloccinum. The following statement was printed in bold letters across the top of its box, "Clinically proven for symptoms of flu. Gentle and effective. No known side effects." I searched the archives of the National Library of Medicine for the source of this claim but did not find any studies of oscilloccinum in treating flu.

Safety is always a concern. Don't equate "natural" with "safe." We need research on every herbal drug sold in this country to determine whether it is effective—and safe.

The failure to regulate herbal production can result in poor quality control and a lack of biological or chemical standardization. As a result, the potency of an herbal preparation you buy may vary from brand to brand. Ginseng is a particularly good example of the consequences of such a nonpolicy. Unless the bottle says "standardized," what it contains is anyone's guess. You'll also find a tremendous variation in the dosage of feverfew, an herb used to prevent migraines; some bottles have too little of the active ingredient to produce any effect, and others contain more than is necessary. Nor is there any way to know whether an herb is in a form that can be utilized by your body; whether the recommended dosage has been tested on humans, animals, or both; or whether it contains any ingredients other than those listed, and if so, whether they have possible side effects. Many herbal preparations have additional chemicals capable of interacting with other medications you're taking, rendering them either toxic or less effective. Some herbs have been found to be contaminated with arsenic, mercury, and lead; others have deliberately (and secretly) been "fortified" with cortisone, nonsteroidal anti-inflammatories, powerful tranquilizers, and other drugs. "Paraguay tea" is a popular concoction from South America made from the leaves of the holly (*Ilex paraguarinsis*). It normally contains caffeine and theobromine. A batch of it recently caused hallucinations, dizziness, agitation, and a host of other symptoms in three families in New York City. When analyzed, the "tea" was found to have toxic doses of belladonna alkaloids.

How herbs are cultivated is also important, especially for those coming from Asia and South America. There's no way of knowing what insecticides or pesticides were used in their production, and how toxic these may be. For all these reasons Dr. Varro Tyler, arguably the best-known advocate of and authority on herbal medicine in this country, says that herbal medicine in the United States is "a minefield of hyperbole and hoax." Even in China, whence many herbs come, there is such chaos in their production that in early 1996 the Chinese government closed several herb factories and stopped issuing permits for new ones. An official of the State Administration of Chinese Traditional Medicine admitted that "there is a lot of fake medicine in the market."

Adulteration of herbal products can cause disability and even death. In Japan, *shosaikoto,* a mixture of seven different herbs imported from China, has been used since 1974 for the treatment of hepatitis and other disorders. Japanese consumers were using it—and spending the equivalent of almost $400 million a year on it—to stimulate the appetite, settle the stomach, and get rid of colds. Recently, *shosaikoto* was reported to have caused ten deaths from pneumonia, and was also found to result in a deadly interaction when taken together with interferon, used in the treatment of cancer, hepatitis, and disorders of the immune system.

Many herbs are sold in this country by mail-order houses, and who knows where they get their products, or how they're produced? Some herbs from Mexico and the Caribbean arrive in this country labeled as veterinary preparations in order to avoid customs inspection. They are repackaged later and sold for human consumption. Some are intercepted, others are not. And don't depend on the FDA to separate the beneficial wheat from the dangerous chaff. Legislation passed in 1994 has left all "supplements," of which there are currently some 20,000—vitamins, herbs, amino acids, and minerals—virtually immune from FDA monitoring. They can be sold without prior testing for efficacy. It's the FDA's responsibility to prove they're *not* safe, and not the manufacturers' obligation to show that they are! The manufacturer need only provide "reasonable assurance" that the product contains no "harmful" ingredients. Manufacturers may not claim that an herb cures or prevents disease, only that they "recommend" it to someone with "whatever." Some of these companies have their own magazines, whose "contributors" write glowing accounts of how some herb or other saved their lives, neatly sidestepping the need for the manufacturer to make any claims that could be challenged by the FDA. Someone simply makes the claims for the manufacturer, who is beyond the reach of the law. This is called free speech. What an incredible piece of lobbying by the health food industry! By contrast, England, France, Germany, and other European countries have established standards for all herbs with respect to dosage, potency, and purity.

Most people ask their grocer or the proprietor of a health food store about an herb but rarely check with their doctor. That's a big mistake. *Always tell your physician about each and every over-the-counter medicine and herb you're taking.* Ask him or her to determine whether it can interact adversely with any of your other medications, especially blood thinners and heart pills. Don't take *any* herb if you're pregnant (some can induce miscarriage) or nursing. Learn as much as you can about any herb you're taking, not only its claimed efficacy, but—more important—its potential toxicity and interaction with other drugs. Begin with a small dose, and take only one herb at a time, not a combination. Look for the words "standard" or "standardized extract" on the container, indicating an international standard of quality. It's a good idea, too, to keep the label handy in the event that you have an adverse reaction.

Let me make it clear that the foregoing discussion is meant to alert you about how best to shop for herbal medications, not necessarily to deter you from taking them when appropriate. It's easy to write off all herbs when you read that some have caused sickness or even death, but remember that thousands of people die every year from approved prescription drugs taken incorrectly or to excess. Nor do I wish to imply that conventional doctors are all honest and that all distributors of herbs are either frauds or dolts. There are many good companies, such as Twin Labs, Nature's Herbs, Rainbow Light, and Source Naturals, whose products are carefully prepared, standardized, and manufactured with quality control. And many upscale health food stores enforce their own quality-assurance measures by very carefully evaluating the products they sell and monitoring the latest reports very closely. But you need to be more careful with an herb than with a prescription drug, because the checks and balances imposed on prescription drugs do not apply to the making or marketing of herbs.

Now let's look at a few of the more widely consumed herbal preparations.

Teas

Scientific studies have documented the many benefits of tea, ranging from the stabilization of blood sugar to easing asthma attacks. Although three-quarters of the world's production is black tea, most health claims relate to green tea. The two kinds come from the same plant but are processed differently. Black tea is fermented before its leaves are dried; green tea is not. Both contain several chemicals that are biologically active. Their polyphenols are said to protect body cells from damage; their fluoride wards off dental decay; tannin is thought to have antiviral and antibacterial properties; theophylline and theobromine dilate the airways. Most tea also contains a small amount of caffeine, though considerably less than coffee.

Why does Japan, with the highest smoking rate among all the developed countries of the world, have the lowest incidence of lung cancer? It's been suggested that this is because the Japanese are also the world's leading drinkers of green tea (all tea drunk in Japan, and most tea in China, is green). Reputable studies suggest that four to six cups a day of green tea will protect against cancer of the lungs, liver, pancreas, esophagus, breast, and skin. Both green and black tea are also associated with a lower incidence of heart disease, probably because their aspirin-like effect reduces the tendency of platelets in the blood to clump together and cause clots.

Herbal "tea" is a different kettle altogether. Unlike "normal" tea, it is made, not from tea leaves, but from cut or pulverized medicinal herbs, and taken internally, externally as a poultice, or in a bath. It can be prepared by infusion (boiling water is poured over the herb and the mixture allowed to stand for a while before straining); by decoction (the herb is first placed in cold water and then brought to a boil for five or ten minutes); or by maceration (the herb is steeped in cold water, and the mixture is allowed to soak for several hours, after which it is drunk either hot or cold).

Almost 400 different botanicals are used to make herbal teas. Some, such as ginger and chamomile, are useful and generally safe. But beware of ephedra (ma huang), which is converted in the body to ephedrine and pseudoephedrine, both of which can increase heart rate, raise blood pressure, and cause nervousness. Avoid herbal teas with other potentially toxic ingredients such as canigre, guarana, maté, fo-ti, and comfrey (discussed below).

Here's a special warning about teas promoted for weight loss or appetite control. They are sold under many trade names, but they all contain some laxative or stimulant. There were four sudden deaths among women who drank such "diet teas" several times a day for one week or more. Although the mechanism of death was not established with certainty, the tea was highly suspect. I know of one pregnant patient who was having continual, debilitating diarrhea. Her doctors couldn't discern the cause; she had not been out of the country, her stool cultures did not reveal any bugs or parasites, and her digestive functions and bowel appeared normal. Then the patient casually informed them that after her examination she was going to the health food store to stock up on more of her diet tea. It seems she had been drinking three or four cups of this herbal tea daily to slow down her weight gain. She never told her doctors about it, because herbs are, after all, "natural." What's so alarming is that this was an intelligent, educated woman who, like most people, simply was not aware that herbs can have powerful medicinal effects. The consumption of these diet teas is so widespread, and their potential consequences are so serious, that an FDA advisory panel has recommended requiring them to carry a warning label or at least list their laxative constituents.

Here are some of the laxatives present singly or in combination in several nationally marketed herbal diet teas:

- *Senna,* the main ingredient in the laxative Senokot.
- *Aloe,* great for burns, but a laxative when taken by mouth.
- *Castor oil*—shades of my constipated childhood.
- *Uva ursi,* whose main biologically active component,

arbuin, is converted in the stomach to hydroquinone, a carcinogen in rats.

You know exactly what you're getting when you buy a box of Senokot or Ex-Lax. The problem with laxative teas is you don't know what's in them or how much. They may also contain more than one active ingredient. One well-known brand has not only senna, but additional "movers" such as orange peel, licorice root, and other herbs. Some diet teas have four times the dose you'd be apt to take when you need a laxative. An occasional laxative or even a glass of laxative tea once in a while won't do you any harm. The danger lies in not knowing that the tea contains a laxative, and then unsuspectingly taking too much of it for too long. Chronic abuse of laxatives, even if unintentional, is particularly dangerous for anorexics, whose nutrition is impaired to begin with; for pregnant women (there are several herbs that can cause a miscarriage); for the elderly; and for the chronically ill—in fact, for anyone to whom chronic diarrhea can pose a threat.

❖ ❖ ❖ The bottom line? Don't drink any herbal tea unless you're sure you know what it contains, and your doctor okays it. Some of these teas are effective, stimulating, or relaxing. Others can be hazardous. My advice is to stay away from them, especially if you're pregnant or nursing. Particularly avoid those that promise to help you lose weight. If weight loss is your goal, then laxatives are not the way to "go."

Alfalfa

Remember when oat bran was strictly for horses, and alfalfa was cattle fodder? Times have changed! Ever since the report that as little as one bowl of oat bran a day can lower cholesterol, it's now become one of the most heavily advertised cereals and a staple in many homes. There's almost as much enthusiasm for alfalfa, whose proponents insist that it relieves allergies, arthritis, morning sickness, ulcers, bad breath (because it contains chlorophyll), poor appetite, high cholesterol, and a variety of kidney and other ailments. Yet I could not find a single reference in the Western medical literature documenting any of these claims!

My son Herb, to whom this chapter is dedicated, thinks alfalfa is great. He sent me a sixteen-ounce bottle of a homeopathic alfalfa tonic. The label says it "relieves daytime fatigue and nighttime sleeplessness." (Does it have a built-in clock that can determine what time it is when you take it, so that at eleven A.M. it perks you up, and at eleven P.M. it puts you to sleep? Many herbs do have seemingly contradictory actions, depending on your physiological needs. So their effect can vary, depending on the circumstances in which they are taken.) Alfalfa is full of calcium, protein, carotene, trace minerals (magnesium, phosphorus, potassium), and a wide variety of water- and fat-soluble vitamins (A, D, E, K, B_1, B_6, B_{12}, C, niacin, biotin, folic acid, and pantothenic acid). It's also very rich in chlorophyll; in fact, it is the main commercial source of chlorophyll. However, it also contains a toxic amino acid, L-canavine, which can severely depress bone-marrow production in humans and thus reduce the numbers of platelets, white cells, and red cells in the blood. There have also been reports that it can activate lupus in people with this disease.

❖ ❖ ❖ The bottom line? There is no evidence that alfalfa is beneficial in any way to humans as a food supplement. On the other hand, there is a very small chance that it can injure bone marrow or aggravate lupus in persons who already have this disease. I'd leave it to the cows.

Echinacea

This one's a winner. Claims made for echinacea are backed by some solid science, although not as much as the hype would lead you to believe.

Echinacea is native to the Midwest and the Great Plains and grows wild on grassland, in open woods and fields. It was by far the favorite herb of American Indians, who introduced it to white settlers. It was applied to the skin to treat bites of snakes or venomous insects, burns, boils, abscesses, and all manner of sores. Today it is also taken by mouth to "stimulate the immune system" and used topically to promote wound healing. It's almost as popular as vitamin C for treating symptoms of the common cold or flu. These beneficial effects of echinacea have been documented in scientific studies both in this country and abroad, especially in Germany, and it is officially approved in many parts of Europe for use as a wound-healing and anti-infective agent. Echinacea apparently gets white blood cells to swarm to areas of infection. These cells are the first line of defense against most infective agents such as bacteria, fungi, and, to a lesser extent, viruses. Echinacea also increases the production of several components of the immune system, notably the T4 helper cells, as well as interferon, a potent antiviral agent. It increases the production of fibroblasts, cells that form healing scar or connective tissue; and it inhibits the formation of hyaluronidase, an enzyme that melts this connective tissue.

The optimal dosage of echinacea has not been established. I prefer a tincture of fifteen to thirty drops added to some water taken every four hours. If you'd rather drink echinacea tea, take no more than three or four cups a day. Many echinacea mavens recommend one-half to one teaspoon of the *standard* extract in a small glass of water three or four times a day. I never know what to do with the capsules, since the content varies so much, so I don't advise taking them in that form. It's best to use echinacea for five days, then stop for two; repeat the cycle for a total of fifteen days, then stop.

❖ ❖ ❖ The bottom line? Echinacea is a safe herbal preparation that may have anti-infective properties and may stimulate the immune system. I'm comfortable using it with, but not in place of, antibiotics for a documented infection. Try it the next time you come down with a cold or the flu.

Comfrey

Comfrey (*Symphytum officinale*) is a loser. Nevertheless, it has fans who swear up and down that it is fabulous when applied topically to skin wounds and poorly healing infections. However, its pyrrolizidine alkaloids cause cancer in rats and are potentially toxic to the liver in humans and animals when taken orally. I believe that the purported beneficial actions of comfrey are overshadowed by its potential harm. It has been banned for internal use in Britain, where its growers and marketers warn that "no human being or animal should eat, drink or take comfrey in any form." It is still widely used in this country, and you will find it displayed in health food stores. I'd stay away.

Chamomile

Chamomile (*Matricaria recutita,* the Eurasian, or wild variety, and *Chamaemelum nobile,* the garden chamomile of Europe and North Africa) is another winner! Everyone loves chamomile, even establishment doctors and their spouses.

The healing properties of the chamomile flower have been appreciated since the days of the ancient Egyptians,

Romans, and Greeks. Of the two main varieties, the Eurasian is more widely used (and cheaper). Both are safe, effective, and nontoxic, with the exceptions noted below; and more than a million cups of chamomile tea are consumed throughout the world every single day—including in my own home.

The name "chamomile" is derived from the Greek *kamai,* "on the ground"; and *melon,* "apple." So "chamomile" is a *kamai melon.* What can this *kamai melon* do for you? The list is almost endless. In Germany, it is referred to as the *Alles zutraut* herb: the herb "capable of anything." A cup of chamomile tea (it has a subtle apple-like flavor) can help you get a better night's sleep; in the beauty parlor, which my wife occasionally visits (she doesn't need to, but goes because she enjoys the company), you may be offered chamomile tea to relax your facial muscles; it settles the stomach and reduces excessive gas; a chamomile gargle will soothe your sore throat; it relieves sore gums and soothes irritated eyes; inhaled chamomile steam relieves bronchial congestion; a chamomile sitz bath relieves piles (hemorrhoids), lessens muscle spasm, and has been said to ease the pain of arthritis; chamomile reduces menstrual cramps; a chamomile bath (brew a large pot of chamomile tea and add it to the bathwater after straining) will calm a restless or irritable child; chamomile ointment moistens dry skin, improves eczema, speeds wound healing, and is great for sunburn, bedsores, diaper rash, and even radiation burns; if you're blond, it will add a golden tint to your hair.

Have any of the qualities attributed to chamomile over the years been scientifically evaluated? You bet. Among other things, it has been shown that topically applied, chamomile neutralizes some of the undesirable by-products that are thought to be responsible for complications in diabetes; it protects the stomach lining against the irritating effects of aspirin and related products; it interferes with blood clotting very much as aspirin does, and may share some of the other protective effects of aspirin; one of its constituents, apigenin, reacts with the same receptors in the brain as do the benzodiazepines (Valium-like drugs), accounting for its relaxing effects.

In making chamomile tea at home, we use chamomile tea bags, not the loose herb. But should you decide to make the tea from scratch, add one-quarter ounce of chamomile herb to a quart of boiling water, stir, cover, and let it steep for about ten minutes.

❖ ❖ ❖ The bottom line? The ingredients in chamomile are biologically active in ways that account for the many benefits described over the centuries. But make sure of the purity of the product you buy. (Most chamomile in this country comes from Eastern Europe, Argentina, and Egypt.) It is an inexpensive, natural remedy that can ease many common symptoms such as insomnia, nervousness, irritability, stomach upset, colic, menstrual cramps, and a variety of skin conditions. Avoid it if you are pregnant (it may relax the uterus and cause miscarriage), or if you are allergic to it or to flowers in the daisy family.

Feverfew

Feverfew (*Tanacetum parthenium*, a member of the chrysanthemum family) is a native of Europe, but grows everywhere in the United States. The name "feverfew" is a corruption of the Latin-derived *febrifuge*—something that "chases away fever." In the early Greek literature, this herb was described as effective against inflammation, swelling, fever, and menstrual pains. It's been hot stuff here ever since British doctors found that it relieves migraine headaches. In the best-known of their studies, nine of seventeen patients with migraine who had been taking feverfew for several years were given a placebo for six months. The other eight continued taking feverfew. The placebo group had three times the number of migraines as the treated patients. Other studies, both here and abroad, have reported similar results.

What is it in feverfew that has this salutary effect on migraine? The consensus is that it's a chemical called parthenolide. The widening and narrowing of arteries in the head that cause migraine are controlled by serotonin, a substance produced by a component of the blood called platelets. Before the onset of migraine attacks, these platelets clump and make much more serotonin, which then triggers the migraine attack. Parthenolide prevents the migraine by interfering with the aggregation of the platelets. Some pharmacologists believe that parthenolide also decreases the amount of prostaglandin secreted by the body (aspirin has the same effect), thus reducing the severity of the inflammation that accompanies migraine. Histamine, the chemical produced in allergic reactions, is also neutralized by parthenolide to some extent. So it's a triple whammy as far as the feverfew is concerned—reduction of serotonin, prostaglandin, and histamine.

Make sure the feverfew you are taking contains enough parthenolide. In Canada, where it has been approved for use against migraine, each capsule must have at least 0.2 percent parthenolide and the label on the bottle must say so. If you've tried feverfew in the past and it hasn't helped your migraine, you may not have been getting enough parthenolide. Take three tablets a day, and stay with it for several weeks or months. It takes that long to work. Once it's had the desired effect, continue it for two or three years. Side effects are rare. Feverfew is a *preventive,* not a treatment. It works in only one patient in three, and it's a long, slow process. But it's worth trying.

Feverfew is said to have other beneficial effects: it alleviates menstrual pain, stimulates the appetite, lessens the symptoms of the common cold, relieves depression, and eases the pain of arthritis. Many people plant it around their homes and patios because the feverfew plant is also an insect repellent.

❖ ❖ ❖   The bottom line? In Canada, feverfew has been officially approved for the prevention of migraine, and it is sold there as an over-the-counter remedy. Make sure that the product you buy is a whole-plant extract with at least 0.2 percent concentration of parthenolide, clearly spelled out on the label. Data for the effectiveness of feverfew against other symptoms such as arthritis are less impressive. You may try it if you want to, but don't expect miracles. Pregnant women, nursing mothers, children under two years of age, and anyone allergic to plants of the chrysanthemum family should not take feverfew.

Ginger

I must know at least a dozen beautiful women called Ginger. They were probably so named because ginger (*Zingiber officinale*) is such a wonderful root, with a long history of medicinal and culinary use. At one time, in China, India, and Japan, ginger was as expensive as gold. Ginger can be taken as a tea or powder, or in capsules. It's widely used in cooking. The next time you're eating out at a Chinese restaurant, order ginger chicken, or a fish cooked in ginger (it goes especially well with cod or red snapper).

The active components of ginger include volatile oils, the most important of which are gingerols and shogaol. As far as its medicinal uses are concerned, it's most widely used for the prevention and treatment of nausea and motion sickness. But ginger enthusiasts will tell you how good it is for the circulation and that it relieves coughs, lung problems, arthritis, stomachaches, and gallbladder disease.

The most impressive evidence for the efficacy of ginger is in the prevention and treatment of motion sickness and nausea. In one research study, volunteers who were spun around until they became nauseated and dizzy responded better to ginger than they did to dramamine, the standard anti–motion sickness drug. Ginger is also effective against morning sickness. However, you should know that there is some question about its safety when taken on a continual basis to control nausea during pregnancy. The concern is that it may cause uterine contractions, which could result in a miscarriage.

❖ ❖ ❖ What's the bottom line? If you become seasick easily, by all means take ginger with you if you're going on a cruise. It has none of the side effects of the usual antimotion medications (fatigue, drowsiness, dry mouth). The usual dose is two or three 500-milligram capsules a half hour *before* the ship sails. You can take an additional capsule or two every four to six hours after you leave port. Once on board, if you prefer the tea, have one to three cups made with two teaspoons of the powder or the grated root per cup. Steep it for ten minutes. The recommended dose of ginger for morning sickness (usually limited to the first trimester) is a 250-milligram capsule three times a day (but check with your obstetrician before using it). Despite anecdotal reports of the beneficial effects of ginger on the heart, intestinal tract, and lungs, I'd stay with the conventional drugs your doctor prescribes for those disorders. Save the ginger for the cruise.

Ginkgo

Don't confuse ginkgo (*Ginkgo biloba*) with ginseng. They're completely different herbs and used for different purposes.

The ginkgo tree is a living fossil, having been around for almost 300 million years. It survived the Ice Age only in China (where it is revered) but now grows virtually everywhere (even in my own backyard). I am told that the only life surviving at ground zero after the atomic blast in Hiroshima was a single ginkgo tree!

Ginkgo is the most popular herb in France and Germany, where more than a million doses are taken every month. The evidence of its efficacy in the scientific literature is convincing. Ginkgo, a potent antioxidant, is a free-radical scavenger; it relaxes the walls of blood vessels and reduces their spasms, thus increasing blood flow, especially to the brain, heart, and legs. This greater blood flow has actually been measured to be as much as 70 percent. If you have neurological symptoms due to impaired blood flow—for example, certain types of hearing loss and tinnitus (noise in the ears and head); or arterial spasm, as in Raynaud's disease (the fingertips become blue after exposure to cold)—ginkgo is worth trying. However, although one dose of ginkgo has been shown to improve short-term memory for hours, I doubt that it can make a significant difference in the treatment of Alzheimer's disease. The optimal daily dose varies somewhat, but I recommend a total of 160 to 240 milligrams daily, taken in two doses. I have seen no reports of any toxicity at these levels. But be patient. It may be at least six weeks or more before you notice any improvement.

Ginseng

The ginseng root (*Panax schinseng; Panax quinquefolius;* Siberian ginseng) is as old as the hills. Various cultures have for thousands of years considered it synonymous with stamina, sex drive, longevity, energy, and appetite. These fantastic claims have resulted in the use of ginseng by millions of fans the world over. It is relatively nontoxic, and you can take it as a capsule, tablet, tea, tincture, powder, or extract. You'll also find it in candies, sodas, and cosmetics. (Personally, I find its taste disagreeable, as do many of my friends.)

There are several different species of ginseng currently cultivated around the world. The major ones are *Panax schinseng,* grown in Asia; and *Panax quinquefolius,* the North American variety. (Siberian ginseng is a related herb, said to be less potent. It is the form favored by Dr. Andrew Weil.) "Panax" and the word "panacea" are both derived from the Greek for "all-healing." The name probably stems from the ancients' belief that ginseng was a miracle herb. It is used mainly to boost energy, enhance sexual vigor, slow the aging process, correct bleeding disorders, retard arteriosclerosis, prevent cancer, delay senility, lower blood sugar, and even lessen the severity of radiation sickness.

How many of these alleged benefits have been documented? The Chinese and Russian medical literature, not always considered credible by Western scientists, is replete with accounts of how ginseng improves athletic performance, enhances physical and mental ability, prevents stress ulcers, fights inflammation and cancer, and lowers cholesterol and triglyceride levels. Pretty good for one herb! Despite considerable skepticism in the West, there are ongoing studies to try to verify these observations.

Traditional physicians in this country doubt most of the claims made for ginseng because, despite all the laboratory data on mice and other animals, there is little if any convincing evidence of any effect on humans. However, at a recent world conference on ginseng, one Swiss manufacturer of natural food supplements reported that middle-aged Swedish men who received ginseng for eight weeks had a measurably greater capacity for physical work than men given a placebo. Some gynecologists have published accounts of ginseng's usefulness in treating the hot flashes of menopausal women who were unable to tolerate estrogen replacement therapy. This is not surprising, because ginseng does contain estrogen-like compounds. Dr. Lawrence Wang of the University of Alberta, in Canada, believes that one component of ginseng may ameliorate the symptoms of Alzheimer's disease and is continuing his research in this area. In Australia, athletes taking ginseng were found to have increased muscle strength and faster recovery times after vigorous exercise.

The major active ingredients in ginseng are steroid-like substances called ginsenosides and panaxosides. Ginseng enthusiasts call them *adaptogens,* substances said to stimulate the immune system and possess antistress properties. This is rather a vague concept, as far as I am concerned.

Since there is no standardized international method for extracting ginsenosides from the root, it's almost impossible to interpret any of the existing research data or to decide what doses of ginseng are effective, if any. It's been a scandal of sorts even in this country, where analyses of ginseng products purchased by mail order or at some health food stores have shown that some samples contain no active ginsenosides whatsoever, while others have very high concentrations. In fact, ginseng varies so much in potency that it is difficult, if not impossible, to decide how much to take of any given brand! That may be why ginseng raised blood pressure in some human subjects and lowered it in others. What's more, although ginseng is a relatively safe herb, it has been known to cause insomnia (never take it at bedtime), diarrhea, skin rashes, nervousness, vaginal bleeding, and painful breasts (the latter two side effects are probably due to its hormone-like action). Finally, there is the question of adulteration. Given the lack of regulation of the production methods for ginseng and other herbs, it's not surprising that batches have been found to be contaminated by a variety of toxins.

If you are taking ginseng, or planning to, buy it from the same source every time, if possible, and stay with one brand. Although it's hard to specify a dose, given the inconsistency of processing, I recommend no more than 100 to 300 milligrams three times a day of the standardized extract containing 7 percent ginsenosides. If you prefer the crude herb, limit it to two grams a day. In any case, keep your doctor informed.

❖ ❖ ❖ Here's the bottom line on ginseng. On the *plus* side:

- Ginseng has few toxic side effects and is relatively safe when pure and properly made.
- It's been around for thousands of years and has gotten some rave reviews.

The greatest *drawbacks:*

- Lack of standardized dosing, so that preparations may vary from brand to brand and batch to batch, and may also be contaminated.
- Some of the claims for its effectiveness have been substantiated in laboratory animals, but there has not been a great deal of proof of efficacy in humans. Several studies are now under way to explore the mechanisms of action of ginseng, and whether it works in humans.

Should you take ginseng? You now have the facts. Decide for yourself.

Hawthorn

The hawthorn (*Crataegus oxyacantha*) is a small tree with a round, bright-red fruit that holds a single nut. Unlike ginkgo, ginger, echinacea, and ginseng, hawthorn is not an herbal household word in this country. Here's how my attention was recently drawn to it.

Some years ago, one of my patients brought her elderly mother, visiting from England, to see me. The mother had high blood pressure, coronary artery disease, and heart failure. Her symptoms were severe enough to affect the quality of her life. My tests suggested that she was not a candidate for surgery, so I prescribed several drugs to lower her blood pressure, increase the blood flow in her narrowed coronary arteries, and strengthen her heart muscle. She returned to England with these medications, and I heard nothing more from her. Two years later, when her daughter came to see me for a checkup, I inquired about her mother. I did so with some trepidation, fearing that she was no longer alive. "Oh, she's just fine," was the reply. "Is she having any trouble getting refills of my prescriptions in England?" I asked. "Not at all. You see, she's not taking them anymore." The daughter explained that her mother wasn't able to cope with all the side effects—urinating all night from the diuretic, getting headaches from the isosorbide (a nitrate drug that dilates the coronary arteries and reduces angina, but which, in so doing, also widens the arteries in the head), and coughing from the ace inhibitor (this drug is very effective for heart failure but often causes a dry cough). The daughter went on: "Also, she doesn't remember things as well as she did when she was younger, so she was often uncertain about which medication to take and when. Anyway, she was advised to stop all of them and take some hawthorn capsules instead." "Do you mean to tell me that a doctor told her to stop her diuretic, nitrate, and ace inhibitor, and replace them with—hawthorn?" I asked incredulously. "No," her daughter replied, "it wasn't her doctor. It was an herbalist." "And how's she doing now?" I asked. "Just fine. She plans to visit me in a few weeks," she answered.

That sparked my interest in hawthorn. It seems that the flowers, leaves, and infusions from this plant have been used for years to control cardiac arrhythmias, strengthen the force of the heartbeat, slow the heart rate, and increase blood flow from the coronary arteries to the heart muscle— in short, everything my own prescriptions for this patient were intended to do. The active ingredients of hawthorn have been shown to contain large concentrations of fla-vonoids, which may in part be responsible for some of its beneficial actions. A study done in Germany in 1953 demon-strated an 83 percent increase in coronary blood flow in patients receiving hawthorn. Another, in 1995, indicated that hawthorn inhibits the production of a certain cardiac enzyme, possibly explaining some of these favorable effects. I would name that enzyme for you, but 3',5'-cyclic adenosine monophosphate phosphodiesterase is too much for anyone to remember.

Hawthorn is especially popular in England, and it has been officially approved for the treatment of heart disease in Germany. Side effects are said to be few. It's considered so safe that it is an ingredient in candies, which kids eat in large quantities without ill effect. Hawthorn can also be taken as a syrup, as tea (two cups a day made from the coarse, dried herb), or in capsules.

❖ ❖ ❖   What's the bottom line? Hawthorn appears to be effective, but most conventional doctors in this country don't have enough experience with it to justify your aban-doning conventional drugs to use it. If and when the neces-sary research has been done, hawthorn may well be added to existing cardiac regimens, and reduce the dosage of conven-tional drugs required.

Valerian

Valerian (*Valeriana officinalis;* garden heliotrope) is currently among the ten most popular herbs in the world. The Chinese have been taking it for thousands of years to help them relax and sleep, and it was regularly prescribed by Hippocrates and Galen for the same purposes. It is the most widely used sedative in Europe. In Germany, for example, it can be found in more than 150 over-the-counter preparations, recommended for both children and adults. A paper in the *British Medical Journal* said of valerian that it is "perhaps the earliest method for treating neuroses." In addition to these "psychoactive" properties, some patients have told me that it relieves menstrual and stomach cramps.

What can you expect your doctor to prescribe when you ask for something to help you sleep? If he or she has the time to sit down and talk with you (something that's become less and less common in this country), your doctor may advise you what *not* to do at bedtime: don't finish your leftover chores from the office or other tasks that stimulate you; avoid sex if it gives you a "high" (that doesn't mean you have to abstain—simply enjoy it in the morning instead); drink a glass of warm milk or have some other natural source of l-tryptophan such as turkey (since l-tryptophan capsules were found to have been contaminated, they can no longer be purchased in the United States). These steps may help somewhat, but not if you've got a real sleeping problem. So the next step is medication. If you ask about melatonin, you will probably be cautioned not to take it on a regular basis, because we're still not sure about its long-term safety; over-the-counter agents, most of which are antihistamines, may cause problems for men with an enlarged prostate. That brings us to the heavy-duty sleeping pills, all of which can leave you hooked. If you need "something," I believe valerian is a reasonable option. Doctors used to recommend it in the era before Valium and other potent sleeping agents. (Don't confuse non-habit-forming valerian with Valium, a totally unrelated—and habituating—synthetic tranquilizer. You're also safer taking a drink with valerian than with Valium, but don't overdo it, because there can be an additive effect between alcohol and valerian.)

Valerian is an herbaceous perennial plant widely distributed in the temperate zones of North America, Europe, and Asia. Although its root has some constituents that stimulate nerve fibers (which is why 20 percent of people who use it experience a high), its major ingredient, valerian acid, has a calming effect on the central nervous system. That's why it's both a tranquilizer and a sleeping aid.

You can make valerian tea by boiling an extract of the root, or you can take it as a tincture—neither of which I recommend. Both forms are effective enough, but their smell and taste are reminiscent of dirty socks, unwashed feet, or very strong ripened cheese. In fact, the aroma of valerian is so unpleasant that it is the main ingredient of "stink bombs." Most people hate the smell, though your cat, will love it and is likely to rub lovingly against your leg when the aroma permeates your house. Take my advice. Give catnip to your cat; and you take the valerian in capsule form. You'll need at least 900 or 1,000 milligrams at bedtime, but you may use up to three times that dose if necessary. And don't be impatient; it takes about an hour to work. Unlike other sedatives, valerian rarely leaves you with a hangover. How long can you continue to take it? Some of my European patients have used it regularly for years without ill effect; but I suggest that you stop after a month or two, because some cases of depression have been reported after prolonged use.

❖ ❖ ❖ What's the bottom line on valerian? There is abundant scientific documentation of its effectiveness and overall safety. It has earned the designation "generally regarded as safe" (GRAS) from the FDA. Other herbs (kava kava, Saint-John's-wort) are said to have a similar sedative effect, without its odor. I doubt that they're as effective.

Saw Palmetto

Saw palmetto (*Serenoa repens*), commonly known as the dwarf plant, has for years been thought to increase libido, renew sexual vigor, and increase sperm production—effects for which all men yearn. The juice from this plant's olive-sized purple berries is what's alleged to do all these wonderful things. But alas, when put to the scientific test, this sexual panacea has not panned out.

Still, don't give up on saw palmetto, because—sexual effects aside—one of the extracts of the berry inhibits or neutralizes testosterone-5-alpha-reductase, an enzyme that contributes to enlargement of the prostate. The less of this enzyme you have, the smaller, or at least the less enlarged, your prostate becomes. This finding could be very important to men who have an enlarged prostate, known as benign prostatic hypertrophy (BPH). A drug called finasteride (marketed as Proscar) also inhibits this prostate-enlarging enzyme. However, it doesn't always work, and while it's safe, it can sometimes reduce libido and sexual potency.

Urologists in this country, following the lead of specialists in Europe who routinely prescribe saw palmetto, have started evaluating it. They have been assessing such parameters as frequency of urination at night; the force of the urinary flow (the larger the prostate, the more it blocks the duct through which the urine flows, and the thinner the stream); and how much urine is left in the bladder after a man thinks he has emptied it. All indicators were measurably more improved by saw palmetto than by a placebo. The advantages of saw palmetto over any drug are obvious: it has none of the side effects, and it costs considerably less.

The following true story suggests, however, that despite the promising results with saw palmetto, it may take some time before the establishment recommends this herb for routine use. After I had reviewed some of the data on this herb, I asked one of my colleagues, who heads a large department of urology, what he thought about it. Well, he wasn't sure; there hadn't been all that much research done on it; he was hesitant to prescribe it because, after all, we did have a drug approved by the FDA (finasteride) that acts much the same way. His entire response seemed rather embarrassed, until I learned, ten minutes into our discussion, that he personally was taking saw palmetto!

I have no hesitation about recommending saw palmetto, because it appears to be as good as any nonsurgical treatment presently available. It has another major advantage over Proscar; in addition to fewer side effects and less cost, it does not affect the level of prostate-specific antigen (PSA). The PSA level, determined in a blood test, is an important marker of cancer of the prostate. One of the drawbacks of Proscar is that it falsely lowers the PSA level, invalidating this test and making it more difficult to diagnose cancer of the prostate. Saw palmetto has no such effect on PSA. Other effective medications are available to help reduce the frequency of urination and to calm an irritable bladder distended by retained urine, but none shrinks the prostate as saw palmetto does.

If you decide to try saw palmetto, look for the words "fatty acid" or "lipophilic extract" on the label. These terms refer to the only fraction of the saw palmetto berry that works. (Other constituents of the berry are not effective. Drink saw palmetto tea if you enjoy it, but don't expect it to shrink your prostate.) The usual dose is 320 milligrams a day, in two doses of 160 milligrams each, morning and night. You won't be able to pee over a fence the way you used to the morning after you've started it: two or three months may be needed for results to become apparent. Stay with it, but continue the other medications your doctor prescribes to relieve your symptoms.

Goldenseal

Goldenseal (*Hydrastis canadensis*) is also known as "yellow root." Once a favorite of the Cherokee Indians and the early settlers with whom they shared their folklore, it was used mainly to wash out an inflamed eye, as a tonic or pick-me-up, and as a dye.

I recently heard about another alleged property of goldenseal. After some get-acquainted chitchat, a new patient wanted to know if there was anything special about combining herbs and "dope." I had no idea what he was driving at until he told me he'd heard that if you're taking an illicit drug, especially heroin, it won't show up in a urine test if you have some goldenseal before turning in the sample cup. He had applied for a job at a munitions factory and needed to have a urine test for illicit drugs. Since he used these substances "once in a while," he had loaded up with goldenseal the night before. To his surprise, he flunked the test and never got the job. He wanted to know how come. Therein lies the truth about a commonly held misconception of goldenseal, and one of the main reasons it's used. Despite street wisdom to the contrary, goldenseal does *not* obscure the presence of any street drugs in the urine.

I'm afraid goldenseal doesn't pass many other tests, either. Although you can still find some goldenseal eyewash around, there are many better preparations for that purpose. Recently, goldenseal has even been touted as an immune-system stimulant, allegedly increasing the production of white blood cells, whose job it is to fight infection. I was unable to find any serious evidence confirming this. Furthermore, if your child happens to swallow goldenseal, it can cause respiratory failure and death (and the toxic dose varies, so I suggest that you consider any amount to be dangerous). I don't believe that goldenseal has a place in your medicine or herb cabinet.

Burdock

Burdock (*Arctium lappa*) is another one to avoid. Despite its long reputation as a diuretic and liver stimulant, I could find no documentation that it has any significant medicinal effect. Moreover, there have been several reports of poisoning by batches contaminated with atropine, a powerful antispasmodic drug. I mention burdock here because there has been a recent flurry of interest in its potential as an anticancer agent. It is alleged to block the growth of cancerous cells and prevent abnormalities in cell chromosomes. Although this may warrant further research, there is no reason at present for anybody to use this herb.

Prickly Ash Bark

American Indians discovered that prickly ash bark (*Zanthoxylum americanum*) is a local anesthetic and used it to alleviate toothache. If you happen to develop a bad toothache far away from your dentist; *and* if you don't have aspirin, ibuprofen, or Tylenol handy; *and* if you're a botanist or can recognize either the northern or the southern prickly ash tree—you're in luck. Just break off a piece of the bark, chew it thoroughly, then wrap the pulp around your aching tooth and leave it there until you can find a drugstore or a dentist. Modern research indicates that some constituents of the bark have antiprostaglandin or aspirin-like properties, which account for its mild analgesic effect.

❖ ❖ ❖ The bottom line? Interesting, but not world-shaking, and hardly a reason for you to rush to your health food store to buy prickly ash bark. There are more effective products. But should you ask your herbalist about it, he or she may tell you that it is also an excellent circulatory stimulant; that it will relieve cold hands and feet (get your thyroid function checked if your feet and hands are cold); improves arthritis; relieves cramps, indigestion, colic, and flatulence; and lowers fever. I can't find documentation for any of these claims. My advice is to stick with chewing it for toothaches when you're lost in the woods.

Licorice

Licorice (*Glycyrrhiza glabra*) has been used over the years as an ingredient in candies because it is fifty times sweeter than sugar. However, you're not likely to find much real licorice in the red and black candy your children (or you) love to chew. Although licorice candy does exist, much of what is sold as a confection contains very little of the root, and its "licorice" taste is due to the addition of anise oil, a member of the parsley family. Licorice also gives tobacco an interesting taste and aroma, and it is often added to medicines to disguise an unpleasant or bitter taste.

The major medicinal action of licorice was discovered only fifty years ago, when a Dutch doctor observed that it promoted the healing of peptic ulcers. To this day, it is widely used for that purpose in Europe, especially in Denmark. (Don't ask me why Denmark. It's just one of those strange facts.) Because of its anti-inflammatory and antiallergic properties, it has also been used to suppress and liquefy the cough of the common cold and ease the pain of a sore throat. From these relatively modest beginnings, researchers have moved on to investigate other potential uses for licorice: to fight cancer and HIV, as a painkiller and an immune-system stimulant; to prevent cavities and dental plaque, and, most recently, to treat chronic fatigue syndrome. Scientists may eventually prove that licorice really does have some or all of these effects, but for the moment it's all speculation. The important fact for you to remember *now* is that even a little real licorice can cause big health problems, because it acts like a steroid, a powerful hormone. An "overdose" of licorice (the amount that can hurt you is unpredictable), whether it's from eating too much real licorice candy, sucking on too many licorice cough drops, or consuming too much of the root while treating your ulcer, can cause retention of salt and water, high blood pressure, potassium depletion, and other hormonal effects. The danger is even greater if you also happen to be taking steroids such as cortisone, heart medications such as digoxin, or water pills (diuretics), or if you already have high blood pressure (hypertension). "Licorice-induced hypertension" is a common, well-documented, and dangerous condition. It's a result of the hormonal action of licorice, which is why naturopaths use it to treat chronic fatigue syndrome (on the assumption that this condition is due to a deficiency of adrenal hormones). Seems a bit far-fetched to me, but even if the theory is correct, why not just give the missing hormone in the conventional way, which allows you to administer precise doses?

❖ ❖ ❖ The bottom line? I don't advise the medical use of licorice for any reason. There are better ways to treat ulcers and the symptoms of the common cold. The rest of the claims made for licorice, even if promising, are premature. The hazards of an overdose are too great, and the alternatives too effective, for you to make licorice the treatment of choice for whatever ails you. There is no truth to the doggerel "Candy is dandy, but licorice is quickerish."

Oil of Evening Primrose

Oil of evening primrose (EPO), whose botanical name is *Oenothera biennis,* is a native American wildflower that was brought to Europe in the seventeenth century. The oil extracted from its seeds is used worldwide for the prevention and treatment of a large number of different ailments. The controversy surrounding EPO is a classic example of how opinions can vary when it comes to herbs, holistics, and health, given the same basic information. Although a large body of data documenting its effectiveness has been published in scientific journals throughout the world, including the United States, the FDA ruled in 1992 that EPO is not generally recognized as safe for human consumption, and it remains an unapproved food additive. I'm not sure the FDA is right. What's more, I predict that if the data now appearing continue to be validated in ongoing studies, this decision will be amended.

In the case of EPO, unlike some other "natural" products, there is a sound and logical theoretical basis for the benefits attributed to it. Let me tell you about them before we go into the claims and the evidence that purports to support them. Evening primrose oil contains more of the essential fatty acids (EFA), called linoleic and gammalinolenic acid (GLA), than any other food. The body does not make GLA; it must be consumed in the diet. The salient fact to remember about GLA and about essential fatty acids in general is that they are constituents of cells and are also the precursors of

prostaglandin, the vital body chemical that fights inflammation. (GLA is so important that it is found in large amounts
in human milk.) EFA deficiency can occur when there's not
enough of it in the diet or if the body is unable to process it
efficiently. Several diseases and symptoms have been attributed to a lack of EFA (and GLA). These include heart disease, obesity, a variety of skin disorders (such as eczema),
infertility, liver and kidney problems, arthritis, and many
more. Replacing the missing fatty acids—and EPO is a good
way to replace them—is reported to have a beneficial effect
on many of these conditions. A Canadian product called
Efamol, which contains a standardized amount of EPO, has
been tested in the treatment of a number of disorders and
has been shown to have salutary effects. For example,
placebo-controlled double-blind studies revealed that EPO
lowers cholesterol by some 30 percent and reduces the "clot-
tability" of the blood much as aspirin does (by reducing the
tendency of the blood platelets to clump together); EPO
inhibits tumor growth when injected into animals; patients
with rheumatoid arthritis required fewer painkillers with
EPO than with a placebo; symptoms of premenstrual syndrome (PMS), such as irritability and breast tenderness, are
improved more substantially with EPO than with a placebo
(a fact to which many of my own patients will testify);
eczema and other skin disorders improve more obviously
with GLA than with a placebo; the nerve disorders that
occur in some diabetics have also been reported to improve
with GLA. Equally important, despite the fact the EPO has
not qualified for the FDA's designation GRAS ("generally
regarded as safe"), there were virtually no side effects from
EPO supplements used in these or in other studies.

More work remains to be done with EPO. For example,
there are no uniformly accepted doses. I would like to see
long-term studies to determine whether the cholesterol-
lowering and antiplatelet effects are indeed translated into

reduced rates of cardiac death and heart attacks. It would be nice to know whether taking EPO over the years has a favorable effect on rheumatoid arthritis in addition to easing its symptoms. Perhaps people prone to cancer could be given EPO and monitored for a period of time to see whether they have a lower incidence of the disease. (Such studies were carried out with beta carotene in heavy smokers vulnerable to lung cancer. Incidentally, to everyone's surprise, the beta carotene was not protective.)

EPO is available in gelatin capsules. They are preferred by most naturopaths. I can't advise you about the dosage. Your best bet is to follow the directions on the bottle you buy.

❖ ❖ ❖   Here's the bottom line on oil of evening primrose. All the data thus far reveal that it contains important essential fatty acids, deficiencies in which can cause a variety of serious ailments, ranging from skin disorders to heart disease. Whether it's superior to existing treatments for these conditions has not been established, but it's certainly more effective than a placebo, and it is well tolerated. If you suffer from any of the disorders mentioned above for which clinical trials have been carried out with positive results, there is no reason not to try EPO.

The foregoing are just a few of the many herbal preparations being sold in stores and mail-order catalogues. The hype that accompanies them is not always reliable. Some are useful; many are not. Several are harmless, regardless of their efficacy; others can be toxic. Learn as much as you can about each and every product that tempts you—*before* you use it. Unfortunately, I could not find any other books on "herbal medicine" currently available, with the exception of those written by Dr. Varro Tyler, that provide an impartial assessment of the substances they describe. It's a good idea to ask around about any medicinal herb you plan to take.

❖ 18 ❖

HIGH COLONICS
AND COFFEE ENEMAS
Public Enema Number One

People have been giving themselves enemas since time immemorial. But did you know that this practice is said to be of divine origin? It was none other then Toth, the ancient Egyptians' god of medicine and science, who introduced the enema to humankind. This is how it happened. One fine summer day, Toth invited himself to a little picnic that the pharaoh's personal physician-priests were enjoying on the banks of the Nile. Now, the Egyptian gods, for some reason, were always wandering about in disguise. On this occasion, Toth assumed the form of an ibis, a sacred bird with a very large beak. After attracting the doctors' attention, he waddled down to the river, where he filled his beak with water. As the assembled medical group looked on, Toth (you'll never believe this) actually inserted the tip of his beak into his own anus, where he discharged all the water. The witnesses of this incredible act—the top doctors in Egypt, the cream of their profession—were perceptive enough to understand the implications and importance of this divine message. They hurriedly packed up their picnic gear and rushed back to the palace, where they promptly proceeded to give a very surprised pharaoh his (and history's) first recorded enema! He must have liked it, because in gratitude, the squeaky-clean king bestowed upon the physician who had administered it the august title "Guardian of the Royal Bowel Movement." Although this decoration is currently obsolete in the few remaining royal courts of the world, we have been giving ourselves (and each other) enemas galore since that fateful day in Egypt! Should we, in fact, be doing this; and if so, under what circumstances?

This nation is obsessed with constipation. Americans believe that they are full of toxins, and that unless the colon is emptied every single day—or, preferably, more often— some terrible fate will befall them. (The same rationale of "purification" was used to justify bloodletting years ago.) Europeans tend to prescribe "cleansing" enemas at the drop of a hat, and even use the rectum to feed people and administer medication. The world is full of enema enthusiasts, many of whom (doctors included) believe that regular "irrigation" of the bowel, regardless of whether it's full, is an absolute "must." For them, a purged colon is the key to happiness and well-being, and essential for the prevention and treatment of disease.

I guess I'm old-fashioned when it comes to enemas. I happen to believe that the colon was meant to eliminate stuff, not to receive it. So I normally prescribe enemas in only a few special situations. For example, when you're constipated and uncomfortable, it's perfectly reasonable to solve the problem with a small enema (or a laxative). You'll also need an enema if you're about to have your bowel operated on or examined. Surgeons insist on a thorough cleaning before they "go in"; so does the gastroenterologist who's about to look into your colon with a scope, and the radiologist who will be studying it with a barium enema. People who have lost the tone in their bowels because of some neurological problem such as a stroke, so that they are unable to eliminate its contents, need enemas regularly. There are also special circumstances when an enema is given to eliminate an excess of some toxic substance—such as potassium, which can accumulate in certain forms of kidney failure. As far as I am concerned, these are the major legitimate uses of the enema. Always remember that you can end up making your colon "lazy" if you subject it to chronic laxative or enema abuse.

You can have your enema in a variety of forms and flavors (but no tasting, please). Soapsuds are effective because they transiently irritate the bowel, causing it to contract. However, prepackaged solutions work just as well and are more convenient. (The Fleet's in!) Some doctors routinely employ additives such as sesame, licorice, and even mixtures of milk and molasses. The coffee enema (I prefer mine black, without sugar), discussed in greater detail below, is widely recommended by practitioners of alternative medicine for the treatment of various forms of cancer.

The *high colonic* is the Rolls-Royce of enemas. It's given by attaching extra tubing to the nozzle, so that water—lots and lots of water, anywhere from 5 to 25 gallons—is introduced far up into the colon. High colonics are usually administered by full-time "specialists" who charge anywhere between $50 and $100, depending on who does the procedure and where (I mean geographically, not anatomically). But don't do it on your own. It's okay to be the captain of your own Fleet, but save the high colonic for the experts.

Is there any rationale for the regular, routine use of the high colonic if you have no symptoms? Does it do any good? Any harm?

Colon therapists, many of whom are naturopaths, other holistic doctors, chiropractors, and acupuncturists, claim that everyone needs "detoxification" to eliminate the poisons—the "slime" and the thick, encrusted stool—that accumulate along the lining of the gut. According to them, this treatment is especially important if you have symptoms of "toxicity" and it will prevent them if you don't. According to the proponents of high colonics, anyone who's constipated is toxic, as is anyone who has pimples or blemishes on the skin, is chronically tired, has trouble sleeping, is overweight, suffers from colitis, or complains of pains in the muscles and joints. That adds up to virtually everyone—including me. But the fact is that the lining of the colon sloughs off and is renewed daily! Nature provides its own "high colonic" without putting you to the trouble, cost, or risk of having it done artificially.

No one has ever identified the mysterious toxin that is the target of the high colonic; I am not aware that any of these therapists has ever performed an analysis of the products of a routine colonic irrigation; I have never observed any differences in blood tests taken before and after a colonic that could serve as evidence of "detoxification." So far as I'm concerned, the concept of detoxification with enemas is poppycock.

The colon therapists also promise to rid you of parasites (worms and the like) that happen to be residing in your bowel. But if you are, in fact, harboring such boarders, there are more effective, more predictable, and safer ways to get rid of them.

So there's no proof that repeated high colonics do anyone any good. But can they hurt you? Although dangerous complications have been reported, the risk is small when they're done by experienced therapists. However, you don't have to be an engineer to understand that repeated irrigation with gallons and gallons of water can stretch the bowel so that it eventually loses its ability to squeeze the stool down and out. When that happens, you've really got a constipation problem. Even more serious is the risk of spreading infection from one person to another if the machine used for the enema is not thoroughly cleaned between treatments. (Bet you hadn't thought about that!) Failure to clean the device adequately resulted in an outbreak of amebiasis and several deaths in Colorado some years ago. Bowel perforation from the nozzle has also been reported in several cases. Because of these and other documented hazards of regular colonic irrigation, and given the absence of proven benefits, this procedure should not become part of your way of life.

The *coffee enema* for the treatment of cancer was popularized some fifty years ago by Max Gerson, a doctor whose anticancer diet is discussed in chapter 14. Coffee enemas remain extremely controversial and are totally rejected by the "establishment." However, they also have many adherents and are still actively prescribed to hundreds of patients every year by Gerson's daughter and her associates in the Gerson clinic in Mexico, and by several other alternative cancer therapists.

Gerson believed that all patients with cancer need to be detoxified. In his view, they have been poisoned, both internally and externally, by food contaminated with insecticides, herbicides, preservatives, artificial coloring, and added sugar, starch, and salt. Gerson was also of the opinion that artificial fertilizers have depleted the soil of many vital protective nutrients. He and others were convinced that tumors also generate toxic waste, which needs to be eliminated; and that an enema, especially one containing coffee, repeated as often as every hour, is the best way to eliminate them. Why coffee? Because it allegedly stimulates the liver to produce more of the bile in which the accumulated toxins and poisons leave the liver, and because it dilates the ducts that carry bile from the liver to the intestine and out of the body. This theory sounds reasonable, but I was unable to find any evidence anywhere that coffee, whether by enema or freshly brewed and drunk from a cup, causes the liver to excrete more bile.

Coffee is also said to activate a liver enzyme that destroys free radicals, the harmful end products of metabolism, wherever they accumulate in the body. Again, I could not find any evidence in the scientific literature that any enzyme is activated by coffee, whether taken by mouth or by rectum.

The coffee enema is also alleged to reduce the pain of cancer, so that patients need fewer narcotics. This frees the liver from the burden of dealing with the toxicity caused by some of these drugs. Although there have been some reports documenting the pain-relieving properties of coffee enemas, these effects appear to be only modest. Most cancer patients I know would rather have an injection to kill their pain than endure hourly coffee enemas. So would I.

Moreover, although coffee enemas are said to promote the excretion of toxins—poisons—from the liver, not a single such "toxin" has ever been identified. So the coffee enema is credited with dilating the liver ducts to excrete more of a substance that we don't even know exists. This reasoning is unacceptable to a scientist. Even if there were such a carcinogen (a cancer-producing material), increasing the production of bile and dilating the ducts that carry it would make little if any difference. That's because 95 percent of all the bile excreted by the liver, in whatever amounts, is reabsorbed and returned to the liver before it ever gets down to the colon for elimination. This reabsorption is something one would not want to interfere with, for bile contains vital ingredients that the body needs, cannot afford to lose, and must recirculate. Enemas every few hours for a period of weeks or months interfere with the reabsorption of these bile salts and can result in severe deficiencies of enzymes that permit the digestion and absorption of fat, fat-soluble vitamins (A, D, E, and K), and calcium. As far as stimulating the liver to make more bile is concerned, drugs such as phenobarbital do that too—again, much more easily and more effectively than enemas.

Gerson also believed that in addition to eliminating dangerous toxins, coffee enemas promote the absorption of vitamin A. This theory is plausible. Vitamin A probably increases the production of interleukin-2, an important natural cancer-fighting substance that potentiates the activity of killer cells. However, the link between vitamin A and coffee enemas remains speculative.

Each of Gerson's theories about coffee enemas has been subjected to scientific analysis. Here are some pertinent conclusions:

- Conventional cancer specialists believe that although innovative fifty years ago, Gerson's concepts are primitive by today's standards—that the modern understanding of the roles of immunology, genes, biochemistry, and nutrition in the causation and treatment of cancer has left Gerson and his coffee enemas far behind. (Why does the word "behind" crop up so often in discussions about enemas?) Much has been learned about cancer since the toxin theory was postulated 100 years ago.
- Perhaps the most telling argument against coffee enemas is that their proponents recommend them for the treat-

ment of virtually *all* cancers, even though researchers believe that cancers have several different causes and mechanisms, and they respond to different drugs and treatments. For example, some cancers shrink after radiation but others don't; some respond to hormonal therapy but others do better with chemotherapy; and so on. It seems simplistic to lump them all together and prescribe an arduous regimen of coffee enemas for the lot.

❖ ❖ ❖   The bottom line? The number of enemas required, day in, day out, for weeks and months to produce the benefits claimed in the treatment of malignant disease is inconvenient at best and a particular hardship for someone with cancer. Enemas can result in nutritional deficiencies and changes in the composition of the body fluid that can even cause death.

Various infections, including amebiasis, have been reported from contaminated machines used to administer enemas.

Enemas should be taken only to address a particular need, such as relief of temporary constipation or preparation of a patient for surgery or for examination of the bowel, and in one or two other special circumstances.

There is neither logic nor proof to justify routine, regular high colonics or an intensive program of coffee enemas for the treatment of cancer or anything else. The toxins that both types of enemas are said to eliminate have never been identified, either in the liver or in the intestines, and their existence remains in doubt.

❖ 19 ❖

HOMEOPATHY

Is Nothing Really Better
Than Anything?

On a recent trip to Paris, I couldn't resist the delicious, gravy-drowned, cholesterol-laden, fat-filled food for which the French are famous and against which I caution my patients. So I indulged recklessly and paid the price—nausea, gas, and bloating. While browsing at a small drugstore near my hotel, where I had gone looking for something to settle my stomach, I saw row upon row of homeopathic pills, powders, and potions. Their labels "guaranteed" a cure for virtually everything from flu to hemorrhoids. There was rhus tox (poison ivy), kalmia (mountain laurel), hypericum (Saint-John's-wort), all manner of kali (potassium) preparations, and on and on. The druggist on duty told me that these homeopathic remedies sell faster than he can replace them, and that French pharmacies, unlike those in America, are required by law to stock them. According to him, one-third of family doctors in France prescribe homeopathic medicines, 36 percent of the French population use them, and eight university medical schools offer a postgraduate degree in homeopathy.

What exactly is homeopathy, and how did it evolve? The term is derived from the Greek *homoios,* "similar" or "like"; and *pathos,* "suffering." Interestingly, homeopathy is one of the few branches of alternative medicine that did not originate in Eastern culture. Hippocrates first observed in the fourth century B.C. that large amounts of certain natural substances can produce symptoms in healthy people resembling those caused by disease, while smaller doses of these same substances can relieve those symptoms.

Two thousand years later, in the 1790s, a respected German doctor, Samuel Hahnemann (after whom the famous medical college and hospital in Philadelphia are named), amplified this concept and transformed it into the practice called homeopathy. Appalled by the enthusiastic bloodletting and toxic medications prescribed in his day, Hahnemann sought a kinder, gentler, more effective way to prevent and treat disease. He tested Hippocrates' theory, according to which tiny amounts of substances derived from plants, minerals, and animals can enhance the body's resistance to disease. He was his own first subject, taking two daily doses of cinchona, whose active principle is quinine, then as now used to treat malaria. Surprise! After several days, he developed the classic symptoms of the disease, thus confirming the first part of Hippocrates' theory. He "went public" with his testing and gave a wide variety of other medications and natural substances to healthy people to see if he could reproduce his observations. He called these experiments "provings." Many of the agents he used did cause symptoms of specific diseases; he further found that he could often treat those symptoms with very small doses of the same agent that had provoked them.

Hahnemann postulated that the microdoses worked by stimulating specific defense mechanisms in the body, and he called this phenomenon the "law of similars—like cures like." Hippocrates had originally put it this way: "Through the like, disease is produced; and through the application of the like, it is cured." In a similar vein, Paracelsus, a famous physician of the sixteenth century, wrote that "sames must be cured by sames."

Hahnemann then went on to formulate his "law of infinitesimals," according to which the more dilute (the weaker) an agent is, the greater its healing power. To find the smallest effective dose of a medication, he produced weaker and weaker dilutions by adding distilled water or alcohol, vigorously shaking the vials to mix the contents, discarding nine parts, and replacing this amount with more distilled water or alcohol, a process called "succussion." He continued the dilution procedure until virtually *no* active principle could be detected in the vial by the usual testing methods. This, according to homeopaths, makes it possible to use ordinarily toxic substances with relative safety to treat disease. The final "potency" of any homeopathic agent is expressed on the label of the preparation by a number after the name of the drug. The higher the number, the greater the dilution.

Homeopathy flies in the face of modern pharmacology and is considered by the scientific community to be absurd, irrational, and helpful only as a placebo. However, homeopathic practitioners insist that their preparations, though pharmacologically inert, are *biologically* active and able to stimulate the immune system. Homeopaths claim to have done experiments showing that the body possesses a "life force," or "vital force," that is sensitive to these submolecular doses. However—as with the *ch'i* cited by acupuncturists—Western scientists have never demonstrated its existence.

Homeopathy does sound a bit odd, but before you dismiss it, think for a moment of vaccination and desensitization. Inoculating millions of people with tiny doses of cowpox—a relatively benign virus structurally related to its cousin, smallpox—eventually wiped smallpox off the face of the earth. Actually, long before this concept was introduced by William Jenner in the 1800s, generations of peasants had observed that rubbing infected cowpox fluid, the secretions from the sores, on the skin of a healthy person enhanced resistance to the disease. The human immune system mistakes cowpox for smallpox, produces antibodies designed to attack it—and good-bye, smallpox! When you're allergic to a particular substance, your doctor desensitizes you to it by repeatedly giving you *tiny* amounts of the offending agent until your body becomes resistant or immune to it. Not too different from the theory behind homeopathy, is it? There are other analogies between homeopathy and conventional medicine. For example, a lower dose of aspirin taken daily is more effective in preventing the clogging of blood vessels than a larger dose. Most doctors prescribe "baby" aspirin (81 milligrams) for this purpose, rather than the standard adult dose (325 milligrams), and some prefer even smaller amounts.

Unfortunately, however, there are flaws in these analogies. For example, vaccines are not rendered more effective by dilution; nor are they natural plant, mineral, or animal substances like those used in homeopathy. What's more, virtually every medication requires a certain minimum dose before it is effective. Just try taking ten units of penicillin instead of the millions needed to cure pneumonia or some other infection!

How do homeopathic practitioners decide which ingredient to prescribe for a particular illness? They refer to the bible of homeopathy, the *Homeopathic Pharmacopoeia,* which was first published in 1897 and is updated regularly. How were the many hundreds of homeopathic drugs listed there discovered and their recommended doses determined? By "provings" done on healthy volunteers, just as Hahnemann did 200 years ago. The homeopathic practitioner is as familiar with these agents (prepared from flowers, roots, berries, vegetables, seeds, salts, snake venom, honey, and the ink of the cuttlefish, to name a few), as your doctor is with his or her pharmaceutical armamentarium. Homeopathic remedies are sold in tablet, liquid, ointment, or granular form, just like conventional drugs, often with sugar added. These remedies were legitimized in the United States (over the strong objections of the medical community) by the Food, Drug, and Cosmetic Act shepherded through Congress in 1938, largely owing to the efforts of Senator Royal Copeland, who just happened to be one of America's foremost homeopathic practitioners.

A homeopathic physician is apt to analyze your symptoms in much greater detail than even the most attentive, unhurried, conventional doctor. An establishment doctor evaluates symptoms in terms of the disease that's causing them; homeopaths, on the other hand, believe that symptoms are patient-specific, not disease-specific. They assess your lifestyle—the environment in which you live, work, and play; your state of mind; your diet; your personality; your family history; and so on. This concept is so complex that some homeopaths now resort to computers to correlate the data they obtain from their patients. It's not unusual for two people with seemingly identical complaints to be diagnosed and treated totally differently by their respective homeopaths.

In most cases, homeopaths prefer to prescribe just one medication to deal with whatever ails you, but they may also use combinations. They believe that we are overmedicated to begin with, and that we need to be detoxified from all the drugs our doctors prescribe. They correctly point out that toxic reactions to conventional medications account for as many as one third of all hospitalizations.

Homeopaths claim that they can relieve or cure virtually every disorder and symptom, including pain, allergies, asthma, arthritis, epilepsy, diabetes, skin rashes, flu, the common cold, fatigue, premenstrual syndrome and other gynecological complaints, backache, headache, and an array of emotional disorders—all without side effects, because the substances they use, though immunologically strong, are pharmacologically weak. Like practitioners in other branches of medicine, homeopaths say that early intervention yields the best results. They also emphasize that in an acute emergency—for example, if you're bleeding to death—you should see a conventional M.D. Under such circumstances, their minimal interventions and tiny doses are not enough.

The bulk of the support for the effectiveness of homeopathy is anecdotal. Dutch researchers recently reviewed 107 studies by homeopathic practitioners, 81 of which reported positive results. The reviewers did not agree with these conclusions; they criticized the manner in which the homeopaths had conducted their research, which, in their opinion, did not meet scientific standards. Still, there is some evidence that homeopathy is more effective than placebos. For example, doctors reported favorably in *The Lancet,* one of Great Britain's most prestigious medical journals, on the outcome of homeopathic therapy for twenty-four asthmatics. All took placebos for one month; then for the next two months half continued with the placebo and the rest were given a homeopathic agent. Neither the patients nor the doctors knew who was getting what. When the results were tabulated, the patients treated homeopathically had a 30 to 40 percent measurable improvement in their breathing, while only 12 percent of placebo patients responded. In another double-blind study published in the same journal and validated by statisticians at the University of Glasgow, patients with hay fever who received homeopathic preparations required only half the dosage of antihistamine needed by patients given placebos. A paper in the *British Journal of Pharmacology* reported that symptoms of influenza responded slightly better to homeopathic drugs than to a placebo. In a report published in the mainstream journal *Pediatrics* in 1994, American doctors conducting a randomized clinical trial of eighty-one Nicaraguan children with diarrhea found that the patients given homeopathic agents had much shorter bouts of diarrhea than those taking a placebo. In an experiment after World War II, soldiers burned by mustard gas responded better to homeopathic agents (greatly diluted solutions of poison ivy, bicarbonate of potash, or mustard gas) than to placebos.

On the other hand, the Norwegian Research Council conducted a double-blind trial of homeopathy in controlling pain in twenty-four adults who'd had impacted wisdom teeth extracted. If you've ever had this kind of dentistry, you know how much it can hurt. First the patients had one wisdom tooth pulled, followed by treatment with the homeopathic remedies arnica, phosphorus, or hypericum. Twenty-seven days later, they had a second wisdom tooth extracted, but this time they received an identical-looking placebo to control pain. There was no difference in effectiveness between the placebo and the homeopathic medication. Another study comparing the effectiveness of homeopathic preparations and nonsteroidal drugs in controlling the pain of osteoarthritis found the homeopathic treatments less satisfactory.

In considering all these results, remember that homeopathy was compared with placebos, not with standard therapy. I know of no scientific evidence that homeopathy is as effective as, or more effective than, established conventional therapy.

Because studies comparing homeopathy with placebos do suggest that homeopathy has some effect, many doctors, including me, believe that additional research is warranted. We must find alternatives to some of our current treatment practices. For example, I worry that many of the antibiotics doctors prescribe are causing resistant strains of bacteria to develop, and that one day these lifesaving drugs may no longer work. This, together with the emergence of more viruses that are impervious to any treatment, makes it imperative that we explore other avenues of therapy—including homeopathy. Homeopathy could be especially important in treating kids. We overmedicate our children, especially with over-the-counter nonprescription drugs. Every year, hundreds of thousands of parents bring their children to emergency rooms because of toxic reactions to decongestants, antibiotics, painkillers, or cough medicines that the children really did not need in the first place. Homeopathic drugs scientifically determined to be safe and effective would be preferable to the more toxic medications now used.

Remember, however, that although *indiscriminate* use of antibiotics can lead to the emergence of antibiotic-resistant bacteria, it's better to use the appropriate antibiotic to treat an infection than to take a homeopathic preparation. (But there is one caveat. Antibiotics should not be used for viral infections, except to prevent the bacterial "superinfection" that often sets in among the elderly and chronically ill.)

❖ ❖ ❖ The bottom line? The medical establishment in this country considers homeopathy nothing more than an exercise in placebos. Still, the establishment more or less tolerates homeopathy—except when it's used to treat life-threatening illnesses for which conventional therapy is known to be effective. The World Health Organization, on the other hand, considers homeopathy a legitimate form of traditional medicine. It is officially sanctioned virtually everywhere in the world, including most of the United States, where there are thousands of homeopathic practitioners—holistic medical doctors, nurses, dietitians, physiotherapists, and other health care workers. Concerned about the cost, side effects, and toxicity of traditional drug therapy, Americans are spending billions of dollars on homeopathic medicines at health food stores and pharmacies, and sales are currently increasing by 27 percent a year. But don't play follow-the-leader. Decide for yourself whether homeopathy is good for you.

My personal recommendation is that you stay with establishment methods that have a proven track record. However, for symptoms that are not life-threatening, and for which conventional medicine has either no treatment or a potentially toxic treatment, homeopathy may be a reasonable alternative. If you decide to go that route, consult a reputable practitioner who is also an M.D. Regardless of the treatment suggested, get a second opinion to make sure that the diagnosis is correct. You can contact the National Center for Homeopathy (801 North Fairfax #306, Alexandria, VA 22314) for more information on homeopathy and the names of practitioners in your area.

If you want to read more on the subject, I recommend *Discovering Homeopathy* by Dana Ullman (North Atlantic Books, 1991); *Everybody's Guide to Homeopathic Medicines* by Stephen Cummings, M.D., and Dana Ullman (Jeremy P. Tarcher, Inc., 1991); and *Homeopathic Medicines at Home* by Maesimund B. Panos, M.D., and Jane Heimlich (whose husband, Henry, developed the Heimlich maneuver) (Jeremy P. Tarcher, Inc., 1981). Don't be surprised, though, if you feel bewildered and overwhelmed—as I did—by the array of products, doses, and treatments these books describe.

❖ 20 ❖

HYDROTHERAPY
Sitz Baths to Sulfur Springs

"Hydrotherapy" refers to therapy using water in any form. Hydrotherapy can be delivered at home, in a hospital, or at a spa. The water can be hot, warm, or cold; in liquid form, or steam, or solid ice. It may be taken internally, by mouth or by any of the body's orifices, or applied externally—in a sauna, shower, bathtub, Jacuzzi, whirlpool, or sitz bath; from a spray or hose; or in a compress, with or without massage.

In my mind, the term "hydrotherapy" conjures up memories of a soothing massage, an invigorating whirlpool, or the leisurely manipulation of a sore joint or muscle by strong yet caring hands. For me, there's no better tranquilizer. But does hydrotherapy have specific medical applications other than reducing stress?

Although most conventional doctors prescribe hydrotherapy for a variety of symptoms, they do not agree with some of the grandiose claims made for it by practitioners of alternative medicine. For example, the Arthritis Foundation endorses hydrotherapy because "soaking in water allows muscles to become relaxed, enabling one to perform a wider range of motion" with arthritic joints; but a holistic practitioner may tell you that it also works wonders for chronic fatigue syndrome and even AIDS.

The granddaddy of hydrotherapy is the water program featured at most spas. Although Ponce de León never did find the fountain of youth, countless people have for centuries been invigorated, relaxed, and rejuvenated—at least temporarily—after "taking a cure" or "taking the waters." Patients often ask me for a "doctor's letter" so that they can go to a spa to have their arthritis or high blood pressure treated and be reimbursed, or deduct the expense from their income tax. I usually give it to them because they do invariably return home more relaxed, a little lighter on the scale, and more limber—their joints less swollen and more mobile. However, although their blood pressure is often lower while they're actually luxuriating in the waters, it almost always returns to its pre-spa level by the time they've come home.

In recent years, the greatest bargains—air fare aside—for such a healthful interlude have been health spas in Eastern Europe: Czechoslovakia, Romania, Hungary, the former East Germany, and now Russia. Some years ago, I visited a spa in what was then the Soviet Union, and although it was bare-bones hydrotherapy in a no-frills setting, my few days there did me a world of good. I enjoyed soaking in the warm waters, I loved the massages, and I participated in the exercise program (although I'm not very physical). I even lost weight—something I haven't been able to do consistently since—not deliberately or because of any diet, but because the food was inedible. Although I was encouraged to join the other guests in their daily ritual of drinking small amounts of the mineral water, its stench of rotten eggs, from the hydrogen sulfide in it, deterred me. My hosts attributed my sense of well-being to the magical combination of sodium, calcium, magnesium, bicarbonate, and sulfur in their particular spring waters. They may have been right, because we are discovering more and more substances that penetrate the skin to exert a medicinal effect. (One of them, capsaicin, derived from hot peppers, lessens skin pain when topically applied.) And my skin did tingle and take on a healthy glow after a bathing session.

Some years later, I moved up a notch on the luxury scale when I stayed at a spa in Italy for a few days. It was similar to the Russian facility—smelly waters, great massage and baths—but much fancier. I gained weight here because of the cuisine, but I nevertheless felt better, more relaxed, and more flexible. The personnel in this spa, like their Russian counterparts, were convinced that the reason I had "responded" so well was the particular composition of *their* natural waters. As in Russia, I was invigorated after soaking in them, even though the chemical composition of the water at the two spas varied considerably.

Although most American spas promise the same invigoration, rejuvenation, and other beneficial effects as the European facilities, they make no special claims for the local water.

Does the composition of "the waters" really make a difference? Do they truly possess intrinsic medicinal properties? Most holistic doctors are convinced that they do; I'd like to believe this, but I'm not sure. I've never seen any scientific studies confirming or refuting these claims.

My own experiences are subjective. I have always found a few days at a spa to be a great experience, a triumph of stress reduction. Any difference of opinion between conventional and holistic medicine concerning the *mechanisms* of the beneficial effects is simply not worth arguing about. I don't really care about the lack of objective evidence that specific ingredients in the water really stimulate the immune system, or improve digestion, or enhance resistance to disease. I don't care to argue whether the sulfur present in some natural springs improves diabetes, controls urinary tract infection, or lessens the severity of rheumatism, or that its bicarbonate reduces allergic responses and aids digestion. There are other proven (though less pleasant) ways to deal with these disorders. The fact is, there is no downside to a few days at a spa for anyone who can afford it, as long as you don't give up proven remedies for any serious health problem.

The expense of a whirlpool bath, a hot tub, or a trip to a spa may be tax-deductible if a traditional doctor gives you a letter saying that you need it, and if you have a generous insurance carrier. But chances are you will not be reimbursed if a holistic practitioner prescribes hydrotherapy for a condition, such as AIDS or chronic fatigue syndrome, for which it is often used but has not been proven effective.

Conventional M.D.s and holistic practitioners both prescribe hydrotherapy mainly as an adjunct to physiotherapy. For example, they apply cold, usually in the form of compresses, to constrict or narrow blood vessels and to reduce blood flow, swelling, and inflammation. An ice pack acts as a mild local anesthetic, and it can alleviate a headache, toothache, nose bleed, sprain, contusion, bruise, or muscle spasm. (But never give an ice pack to someone who has Raynaud's disease, in which the small arteries are sensitive to cold and go into spasm when exposed to it.) Heat, on the other hand, relieves pain by dilating blood vessels and increasing blood flow. The warmth of a heated pool, together with its massaging effect and the buoyancy it provides, relaxes painful joints and weak muscles so that they can be exercised and strengthened. The areas most responsive to such therapy are the neck, shoulders, middle back, lower back, thighs, and feet.

Here are some variations of hydrotherapy and the specific disorders for which they are prescribed by both "camps."

Hyperthermia

Many organisms—bacteria and viruses—find it hard to thrive or even survive in a hot environment. So the body attacks them with fever. Doctors sometimes mimic this natural response by using heat as therapy for a variety of diseases. Heat might be administered in a hot tub or a deep hot bath (at 103 to 104 degrees Fahrenheit), as a hot blanket pack, in a steam room, or in a sauna (for as long as sixty minutes per session). Heat is such a powerful dilator of blood vessels that doctors administer it as carefully as they would a drug. Before the advent of penicillin, hyperthermia was an accepted therapy for several infections, notably syphilis. In addition to retarding the multiplication of infectious agents, fever also increases the production of antibodies, as well as interferon, an antimicrobial protein derived from the white blood cells. Although some conventional doctors use hyperthermia to treat cancer, it is not widely employed by oncologists (cancer specialists).

Some holistic doctors claim that standing upright in hot water to the neck, several minutes every day for six months, will relieve the symptoms of chronic fatigue syndrome. They also allege that when you're vertical in a pool, regardless of the temperature, the pressure gradient of the water forces fluid out of the lymphatic system into the bloodstream, where it expands and enriches the gamma globulin content. In my opinion, this is way, way out, and without any proof whatsoever.

Doctors are very cautious about giving hyperthermia to the very young or the elderly, since people at both ends of the age spectrum are sensitive to elevated temperatures. The same is true for persons with heart trouble, high or low blood pressure (because heat raises the heart rate), diabetes, or multiple sclerosis, and for women who are pregnant.

Doctors may also use *contrast* hydrotherapy, switching from a hot bath or shower to a cold one. The heat dilates the blood vessels, and then the cold constricts them. Some conventional (and holistic) practitioners believe that this sequence invigorates the circulatory system, relieves muscle spasm, and increases resistance to disease.

Whirlpool

This is an excellent form of physiotherapy to rehabilitate injured, weakened, or diseased muscles, especially after a stroke, and to treat paralysis due to any cause. There is no debate about the usefulness of whirlpool hydrotherapy.

Sitz baths

Sitz is German for "sitting," and in a sitz bath you do sit, or immerse your hips in a tub, or bathe your bottom in a bidet at temperatures up to 110 degrees Fahrenheit. (The water should reach the level of the navel—not easy to do in a bidet.) Sitz baths are recommended by every discipline of medicine for a variety of ailments and inflammations of the nether parts of the body, including hemorrhoids, anal fissures, problems with the perineum (for a woman, this is the site of the episiotomy during childbirth), painful testicles or ovaries, vaginal irritation, prostatitis, colitis, lower abdominal pain due to inflammatory bowel disease, diverticulitis, and menstrual cramps. Stay with it for at least fifteen minutes.

You can also try a cold sitz bath (go ahead, I dare you) if you are impotent (no guarantee from me about this one), if you are constipated (there are easier ways to move your bowels), or if you have a vaginal discharge (brrr)—but not if you have a urinary tract infection. You can also apply contrasting heat and cold in the sitz bath. For this, you'll need two tubs; spend three or four minutes in the hot tub first, then only one minute in the cold tub. Repeat this five times, ending with the cold one. Why end with cold and not heat? Beats me, but that's the conventional wisdom.

Ice packs

If you've hurt yourself, or have acute muscle strain or spasm, tendinitis, or an inflamed joint, ice is the way to go. Apply it as often as twenty minutes every hour for the first day or two following the injury. After that, you'll need no more than three sessions daily. Some physiotherapists recommend alternating hot and cold packs—again, always ending with the cold.

Varicose veins

If your legs hurt because of varicose veins, cool compresses will ease your discomfort.

Sciatica or back pain

The discomfort of sciatica or a backache can be relieved by conventional physiotherapy, with emphasis on water exercises in a warm pool, followed (or preceded) by hot moist packs to the lower back. Acute pain should be treated first with ice packs for a few days, then with hot-water packs.

Chronic headache

An ice pack on the forehead or the back of the neck, or a cold shower with the water running over the head, feels good when you have a headache. Some people prefer a hot moist towel on the back of the neck. But for migraine, you'll get more relief by applying alternating hot and cold compresses to the painful area.

Acne

There are several orthodox methods of treating acne, ranging from various creams and lotions to antibiotics and Accutane (but not if you're a woman of childbearing age, because Accutane can produce birth defects). Some dermatologists recommend simply sponging the skin gently with cold water.

Diarrhea

If you develop the runs when you're away from home, without access to Kaopectate, Lomotil, or Imodium, a very cold compress or an ice pack to the lower abdomen or back for ten to fifteen minutes every hour may tide you over, or at least slow the runs down to a crawl.

Athlete's foot

There are several effective over-the-counter creams, powders, and ointments for treating athlete's foot, and there's not much difference among them. But if you soak your feet in warm salt water for ten minutes before applying any of these medications, they will all penetrate the skin more effectively.

Asthma

This is not the kind of illness you associate with athletes, yet one of my sons who was a "wheezer" qualified for his college swimming team. Hydrotherapy in the form of swimming is an excellent therapy for asthma. The breaststroke, in particular, strengthens the muscles of the chest and improves lung function. Remember always to take the medications necessary to prevent asthmatic attacks, and carry with you those that will terminate an attack.

Bronchitis and emphysema

When your air passages are infected, either acutely or chronically, and you're coughing, spitting, wheezing, and always short of breath, antibiotics, expectorants, and drugs that liquefy the sputum will help. (I'm assuming that you've stopped smoking.) To relieve the cough, holistic doctors also often recommend cold-water packs or compresses to the chest, and hot-water packs between the shoulder blades. Try it, especially if drugs don't do the job.

❖ ❖ ❖ The bottom line? Using water to prevent and treat disease is as old as the hills. Hydrotherapy has its adherents in both conventional and alternative medicine; no one has a monopoly on its indications or use. The fundamental difference between the orthodox practitioner and the complementary physician is that the latter makes grander claims for hydrotherapy. However, this is an area that is so safe and so potentially useful that—regardless of the theoretical disputes between the two camps—you should not hesitate to try any form of hydrotherapy that's suggested for whatever ails you.

❖ 21 ❖

HYPNOSIS

Beyond Svengali

What do you know about hypnotism? For example, which, if any, of the following scenarios do you consider plausible?

- A man with no previous criminal record is arrested trying to rob a bank. In his defense, he insists that he was in a "hypnotic trance" at the time and was simply "carrying out orders." He names the hypnotist, who admits that he had indeed hypnotized this man at the time but vehemently denies having instructed him to perform any crime. Leaving aside which of the two is telling the truth, can a hypnotized subject be made to perform any act that is contrary to his or her moral standards?
- A woman has been a chain-smoker for twenty-five years and desperately wants to stop—but can't. She is referred to a hypnotist and, after only one session, never smokes again. Could this possibly be true?

- You see someone at a cocktail party whom you knew many years ago. You remember her as a serious, no-nonsense, successful executive. As you extend your hand in greeting and say, "Hi, there," she stares at you for a moment and then begins to cluck like a chicken! You laugh, sharing the humor with her, but she continues to cluck, even as you try to talk to her. Embarrassed, you excuse yourself. She moves on to speak with someone else, to whom she does not cluck at all. A few minutes later, she seeks you out and explains that some time ago, she was hypnotized at a party and told that after she "awakened," she would cluck like a chicken whenever anyone said "Hi, there" to her. This, she explains, is "posthypnotic suggestion." Is such a scenario possible?

You will find the answers to all these questions further along in this chapter.

The first demonstration of hypnosis I ever saw was at a high school party, long before I became a doctor. The subject, a friend of mine, was a quiet, intelligent, serious young man; the hypnotist was an extroverted accountant. After my friend entered the hypnotic trance, he lost many of his social inhibitions. For example, although he was normally painfully shy, he now sang lustily, danced with abandon, and recited poetry with gusto, all on command by the hypnotist. When he was told that the room was very hot (it was not), he began to perspire; when informed, moments later, that the temperature had dropped suddenly (it had not), he shivered. I was impressed and amused by this display, but it never occurred to me then that hypnotism was anything more than a highly entertaining theatrical stunt.

My second encounter with hypnotism took place at a vaudeville theater a few months later. A frail, elderly woman, randomly selected from the audience, was given two thirty-pound weights to lift. She could barely do so. But after she was hypnotized and told that she was very strong, she began tossing the weights around as if they were made of papier-mâché.

When I entered medical school several years later, the only reference to hypnosis I ever came across throughout the four-year curriculum was a brief historical review in a psychiatry course. There was not a word about how, when, or why I might use hypnosis as a physician. Medical education in those days focused on "straightforward" subjects—how to listen to a heart, remove an appendix, or interpret an electrocardiogram. There was no time to dabble in the "occult." Fortunately, my profession now seems more receptive to investigating and sometimes even applying some concepts formerly labeled fads. That includes a renewed interest in the therapeutic potential of hypnosis.

Hypnotism was formally introduced in the late 1700s by a German doctor, Franz Mesmer (that's where the word "mesmerize" comes from), who claimed that he could cure several kinds of nervous disorders with it. He believed that he could transfer magnetism from his own body to his patients by using iron rods and magnets to enhance the flow. This resulted in a redistribution of the body fluids, accompanied by a "hypnotic trance."

This all sounded a bit weird to Mesmer's contemporaries, who, for the most part, considered him either a charlatan or just plain crazy. Although it did capture the imagination of many novelists who had a field day describing how evil Svengalis would hypnotize an innocent virgin in order to "have their way" with her (an inaccurate connotation that persists to this day), hypnosis was not used medically for years. Then, just before the advent of anesthesia, some observant doctors noted that they could control their patients' pain during surgery by means of hypnosis, instead of restraining them or making them drunk. Hypnosis was used for this purpose for several years until the introduction of ether anesthesia. After that, hypnosis was for the most part abandoned, except by a smattering of psychiatrists, psychologists—and extroverted accountants.

But hypnotism has now come into its own, despite persistent stigmatization because of its identification with Svengali, black magic, and theatrical entertainment. Trained health care professionals, both "conventional" and "unconventional," are using hypnotherapy to treat a variety of physical and emotional disorders. Although the subject is still not formally taught in most medical schools (neither was nutrition, until quite recently), a section on hypnosis has been established at the College of Physicians and Surgeons of Columbia University. It is directed, not by a psychologist or psychiatrist, but by a surgeon who teaches doctors how to hypnotize patients who cannot safely tolerate general anesthesia because of severe lung disease or other conditions.

No one knows for sure how hypnosis works. Many scientists believe that, like the placebo response (see chapter 2) or acupuncture (see chapter 4), hypnosis activates nerve pathways in the brain that cause the release of natural morphine-like substances called enkephalins and endorphins. These "opioids" modify behavior, the perception of pain, and a variety of subjective symptoms, perhaps through the immune system.

Although hypnotized subjects appear to be asleep or unconscious, they're really not. On an electroencephalogram (a recording of brain activity), their brain waves reveal a pattern of profound relaxation completely different from those seen during sleep. Even in this relaxed state, subjects are intensely focused and able to concentrate on what they are told to do. Although hypnosis renders subjects highly suggestible, they are by no means "at the mercy" of the hypnotist. Believe it or not, in a legitimate treatment setting, they are actually very much in charge and are using the therapist to help themselves control their pain, stress, phobias, troublesome habits, headaches, allergies, asthma, skin disorders, and other ailments.

Ninety percent of us can be hypnotized if we want to be and if we trust and have confidence in the therapist. Being intelligent and imaginative helps too. The idea that only the weak-willed can be hypnotized is a myth. In fact, the more motivated you are to take charge of your health problems, the easier it is for you to be hypnotized. A drink or a tranquilizer just before the session may increase the chances of success, at least the first couple of times, but it's not necessary in most cases.

Herbert Spiegel, a doctor in New York City who is a well-known hypnotist, claims that he can predict whether or not someone can be easily hypnotized. Here is how he pretests his subjects: he has them roll their eyes back as far as they can and lower their eyelids at the same time. The more white there is when the eyes are half-closed, the greater the ability to be hypnotized. So if you're considering hypnosis but aren't sure whether you're a suitable candidate, ask a friend to tell you what your eyes look like after you've rolled them up and half-closed them.

Hypnosis was approved by the AMA as a therapeutic tool more than thirty years ago, but its use isn't restricted to doctors, psychiatrists, or psychologists. Anyone who has a mind to do so is legally permitted to hypnotize a willing subject; neither special training nor a license is required. So don't worry if you're caught putting someone into a trance. You will not be charged with practicing medicine unlawfully.

• • •

Hypnosis can be performed in several different ways, all of which are quite simple. In the most widely used method, the subject is asked to track a moving object (such as the famed pocketwatch) back and forth, back and forth, while the therapist monotonously but authoritatively drones on that the eyes are getting heavier and heavier, and that soon they will be unable to remain open. Despite your closed eyes, and all the trappings of sleep, you will actually be focusing very intently on the therapist's instructions. Instead of having you stare at a moving object, some therapists ask you to concentrate on their voice; others may tell you to count backward slowly from twenty or thirty to zero. Whatever the technique, most subjects "go under" within fifteen minutes. After several sessions with the same hypnotist, you can often by hypnotized almost instantly by a key word or a snap of the fingers.

There are various stages or depths of hypnosis. When you are under "lightly," you won't feel any discomfort when pinched or pricked with a needle. But it takes a "deeper" hypnotic state to control severe pain, such as that due to cancer, surgery, and some dental procedures.

Whatever its depth, hypnosis does affect your judgment and perception; for example, you can be more easily convinced of something that is quite illogical. But a professional hypnotherapist would not want, and indeed would not be able, to make you do something that was contrary to your deep-seated values or religious principles. That's the answer to the first question I posed at the beginning of this chapter about the man who was caught robbing a bank. Even during a trance, he would be most unlikely to follow an order to steal—unless, deep down, he really wanted to.

If you're wondering how long you'd remain in a trance if anything happened to your hypnotist, I can assure you that in such an unlikely circumstance, left to your own devices, you'd simply lapse into a deep sleep, awaken refreshed, and probably not even remember that you'd been hypnotized.

Though seemingly in a "trance," a hypnotized subject walks and talks normally and can recall long-forgotten events. Every time you are engrossed in a book, movie, or play, you are, in a sense, self-hypnotized. I've never been "under" myself, but the other day I realized what "heightened suggestibility" must be like. My wife and I went to see the opera *La Bohème*. In the last act, Mimi lies dying, with her distraught lover sobbing uncontrollably at her side. We've sat through this scene many times; we know how it's going to end; we also know it's only make-believe. But every time we see this opera, the lights are dim, the music is beautiful, and we're so totally immersed in what's going on *now* that we cry along with the grieving Rodolfo. We are, in a sense, "hypnotized."

The most important aspect of hypnosis, as far as I am concerned, is that it permits you to manipulate body functions over which you normally have no control. For example, on command, you can increase or slow your heart rate, raise your temperature, alter your blood pressure, perspire, or develop gooseflesh. These responses are all regulated by the autonomic (involuntary) nervous system. The potential for treating high blood pressure, cardiac rhythm disorders, and stress by means of hypnosis is obvious. Under hypnosis, you can also be made to hallucinate—see and hear things that aren't there. You can also relive past, painful experiences buried deep in the subconscious and perhaps now view them from a different perspective—one you can live with more easily.

To end a session, the hypnotist orders you to awaken and tells you how well you will feel. Most subjects feel alert right away, but some are a little drowsy for a few hours.

Then there is the phenomenon of posthypnotic suggestion, in which you are told what to remember, what to forget,
and what specific acts to perform on a given signal *after* you
"awaken." Such instructions, if repeated and reinforced
often enough, can lead to long-term behavioral changes—a
revulsion against tobacco or certain foods, amnesia for an
unpleasant emotion or experience, and even the ability to
ignore pain.

The results of posthypnotic suggestion can be quite dramatic. Some thirty years ago, I referred a patient, then in
her fifties, for hypnosis because she had been smoking two
packs of cigarettes a day since her teens. She quit after
just one session and never smoked again—and she is now
eighty-two years old! That's the answer to the second question I asked at the start of this chapter. But in all fairness,
even though a dramatic result such as this can occur after
just one session of hypnosis, it's really quite unusual. I
recounted this story only because I witnessed it firsthand
in one of my own patients. Posthypnotic suggestion of the
trivial sort, such as being told that after you "awake" you'll
cluck like a chicken every time someone happens to utter a
particular word or phrase, will not last beyond the duration
of the party, and you may not even do it if you really hate
the idea. In any event, it's not the kind of instruction a therapist (as opposed to an entertainer) is apt to give you. That's
the answer to the third question I asked at the beginning of
this chapter.

When it is done for the right reasons by a trained therapist,
hypnotism can be effective, doesn't hurt, isn't invasive, and
doesn't require expensive equipment or drugs. Perhaps most
important, you can do it yourself. Although there are books,
videos, and audiotapes that teach self-hypnosis, you're better off learning it from a qualified health professional. I sug-

gest that you ask your own doctor to recommend one. If he or she can't, contact the American Society of Clinical Hypnosis (2250 East Devon Avenue, Suite 336, Des Plaines, IL 60018) for the name of a practitioner with good credentials in your area.

If you decide that you'd like to try self-hypnosis, there are several techniques. To do it effectively, allow between thirty minutes to an hour. The first step is to relax completely. Sit in your favorite chair, make yourself as comfortable as possible, and let every muscle in your body go limp. Pick an object high in your line of vision—a design on a curtain just below the curtain rod, a volume on the top shelf of your bookcase, or an unlit lightbulb. Concentrate on it, and breathe slowly and deeply as you do. Keep telling yourself how relaxed you are, and after a few minutes convince yourself that your eyes are heavy and that you want to close them. Repeat over and over again a word or phrase, such as "deep, deep" or "very calm"—anything that comes to mind. Now, fantasize a peaceful scene: the seaside, a meadow, a tree, or a flower. Try to generate sensations of numbness, tingling, warmth, coolness, or heaviness in your arms, neck, back, legs, or face. As you continue this imagery, you will gradually slip into a hypnotic state. Once there, tell yourself, just as a hypnotist would, that some part of your body is totally without sensation. Prick it with a needle, or pinch hard. Chances are you won't feel it!

To end a self-induced hypnotic state, count slowly from ten to zero. At the same time, tell yourself that you're becoming more and more alert, and that you will "awaken" feeling refreshed and well. That's all there is to it. But don't expect to become an expert overnight. It takes months of practice and training, but it's well worth the effort. The next time you're in the dentist's chair, or you're in panic about tomorrow's final exam, or you have a sinking feeling when called upon to "say a few words" in public, hypnotize yourself beforehand. No one will know, and you'll be able to tolerate the worst your dentist can do to you; you'll pass your test with flying colors, and you'll probably give the best public speech ever.

Here are some problems that hypnosis has been documented to help:

Asthma

Hypnosis can either prevent asthmatic attacks or reduce their severity, especially in people who are anxious and can be easily hypnotized. Objective tests of the flow of air in and out of the lungs in such cases reveal as much as 75 percent reduction in the irritability and spasm of the air passages.

Pain

Deep hypnosis is more effective against pain than placebos, simple relaxation, or distraction, and it is used by some cancer doctors and physical rehabilitation specialists (physiatrists) for that purpose. It can also reduce anxiety, fear, and muscle spasm, and result in increased mobility of injured limbs and joints. In Parkinson's disease, it can lessen tremor and rigidity. Symptoms of multiple sclerosis, cerebral palsy, rheumatoid arthritis, and paralysis due to strokes or injury to the brain and head can also respond to hypnosis.

Irritable bowel syndrome

About 15 percent of the population, and about half of the patients who consult gastroenterologists, suffer from irritable bowel syndrome (IBS). They have abdominal pain, cramps, diarrhea, or constipation, regardless of what they eat or drink. IBS is notoriously difficult to treat, and people with IBS are often labeled neurotic. Several studies have reported successful treatment of IBS with hypnosis after all other intervention failed. That's not surprising, because the motility of the gut is under the control of the autonomic nervous system, which can be influenced by hypnosis.

Nausea and vomiting

Hypnosis can reduce nausea and vomiting, especially when caused by anticancer drugs. Patients who require chemotherapy over a period of weeks or months may become "conditioned" to feeling sick and nauseated by it. They often awaken nauseated on the day they are due for the therapy, or they become nauseated even before leaving home for the clinic. Such "anticipatory" illness can often be prevented by hypnosis.

Morning sickness

Morning sickness does not generally require treatment. However, there is an uncommon condition called hyperemesis gravidarum (it occurs in fewer than 1 percent of pregnancies), in which severe nausea and vomiting occurs as often as fifteen times a day. The resulting dehydration and malnutrition can lead to hospitalization and threaten the pregnancy. Hypnosis can be extremely helpful in such cases. Ask your doctor about it.

Labor

Pregnant women who are hypnotized or hypnotize themselves have a shorter labor, less pain, and easier deliveries.

Some cesarean sections are being performed under hypnosis without anesthesia.

Phobias and compulsions

Hypnosis can help you deal with your phobias and bad habits—fear of flying, grinding your teeth while asleep, compulsive hair pulling and nail biting, chewing the lips, smoking cigarettes, drinking, taking drugs, or overeating. However, the outcome in these areas is not very impressive. If you want to try hypnosis to stop smoking, for example, you should know that the success rate is no higher with hypnosis than with any of the other techniques used—none of which is anything to write home about. That's because cigarette smoking is more than a dangerous habit; it's an addiction. Still, hypnosis is worth a try.

Conversion hysteria

Hypnosis is especially effective in a psychiatric disorder called "conversion hysteria"—not as therapy but as a diagnostic tool. Patients with conversion hysteria believe, for instance, that they are unable to move an arm or a leg, and this "paralysis" is sometimes difficult to distinguish from that caused by a stroke or a physical injury. The difference between the two is that "hysterical" paralysis disappears during the hypnotic trance; true paralysis remains.

Overweight

Permanent weight loss is one of the most difficult objectives for countless people, however well motivated. I have several patients who have been able to take the pounds off and keep them off. But this demands a lifelong commitment to diet and exercise, which not everyone can maintain. That's why weight control is such a frustrating experience for the great majority of us. Statistically, hypnosis is as effective in weight reduction as most other forms of treatment—but that's not saying much. In most cases, subjects regain the lost weight after six months. Every weight-reduction technique with which I am familiar, including hypnosis, is ineffective over the long term because there are metabolic and chemical mechanisms within the body designed (and determined) to keep us fat. After you start losing weight, no matter how you do it, your body metabolism slows, you burn less energy, and eventually you stop losing and start to gain again.

Stress

Most doctors believe that "stress," depression, and chronic anxiety lower resistance to disease—whether it's infection, cancer, hardening of the arteries, or high blood pressure. Reducing stress by any technique, including hypnosis, should theoretically have a favorable effect on the course of these conditions. However, I have never been convinced of this. Most of the examples of success are anecdotal. There is, however, one study now being conducted in which weekly hypnosis sessions do appear to prolong survival in women with breast cancer. Further studies are warranted.

Bed-wetting

Bed-wetting is not necessarily abnormal before the age of four. However, if it persists beyond that age, the child should be carefully examined to make sure there is no underlying physical reason for it, such as a urological problem. Emotional support, tolerance, motivational counseling, and bladder-stretching exercises—and, above all, patience—are usually the only treatments necessary. But if these measures don't work, try hypnosis. Karen Olness, a doctor at George Washington University Hospital in Washington, D.C., reports that 75 percent of the children, ranging in age from four and a half to sixteen, to whom she has taught self-hypnosis have been able to cure their bed-wetting.

Allergic reactions

Allergic symptoms are caused by the overstimulation of the immune system when you touch, eat, or inhale something to which you are allergic. Exposure to this foreign material (allergy) results in the increased production of antibodies that, in turn, causes your body to turn out large numbers of "mast" cells. These release a chemical called histamine, which is responsible for the itching, sneezing, wheezing, and tearing eyes typical of an allergic attack. (That's why *anti*-histamines are so effective in treating allergic symptoms.) When exposure to an allergen is overwhelming, the resulting symptoms can cause shock (anaphylaxis) and sometimes even death. Since the severity of an allergic response can be modified by mental processes, hypnosis can often reduce these symptoms. This has repeatedly been shown in controlled scientific experiments. I was especially fascinated by one study in which after subjects were injected in both arms with an allergenic substance, the reaction could be aborted in one arm by hypnotic command, leaving the other one red and swollen.

Warts

Warts can become smaller and even disappear in as many as 55 percent of hypnotized children. (Adults, in whom warts are much less common, do not respond as well.) In these cases, hypnotism is assumed to act on the immune system, which contains various blood cells that go by such names as "helper" cells, "killer" cells, "suppresser" cells, and several others. In a series of experiments at the Minneapolis Children's Medical Center, subjects shown a video of these different cells and how they work were able to shrink their warts by increasing the number of some of the cells, and reducing the concentration of others, under hypnosis.

❖ ❖ ❖   Here's the bottom line:

- Hypnosis is a useful medical tool with great potential when performed by trained health providers such as physicians, psychiatrists, and psychologists.
- The common perception that only the weak-willed can be hypnotized is a myth. The more intelligent and imaginative you are, and the more determined you are to participate in your health care, the more hypnotizable you will be.
- Hypnosis is a state of intense, focused concentration, not a form of sleep.
- Hypnotized subjects are not "at the mercy" of the hypnotist, nor can the hypnotist's will dominate them. You cannot be made to engage in any activity that goes against your "moral grain."
- Bodily functions such as heart rate and blood pressure not normally under voluntary control can be altered during hypnosis. This has practical application in the management of several cardiovascular conditions.
- Most people can be taught to hypnotize themselves in order to reduce anxiety, break bad habits, control pain, overcome phobias, and make an addiction easier to overcome, but they should always receive supportive psychotherapy and ongoing reinforcement with other behavior modification techniques.

• Some of the medical areas in which hypnosis has been shown to be effective include: alleviation of asthmatic attacks and other allergic reactions; terminating bedwetting; as anesthesia in dental, obstetric, and other procedures; relieving irritable bowel syndrome; minimizing the nausea and vomiting induced by cancer chemotherapy; reducing stress; managing certain psychiatric disorders; curing warts.

❖ 22 ❖

IRIDOLOGY

Do the Eyes Have It?

The practice of iridology is based on the assumption that a trained observer can diagnose and predict disease by examining the iris (the colored portion) of the eye. The eye is a font of information for conventional doctors, who look at the whole eye, however, not just the iris. For example, the shape and size of the pupils and how they react to light, the color of the sclera (the white portion), the interior of the eye as viewed with an ophthalmoscope, the eyelids, and the movements of the eye can all aid in the diagnosis of many conditions—from high blood pressure, diabetes, and stroke to infections such as tuberculosis and bacterial endocarditis. Ophthalmologists, however, do not consider the iris to be particularly important in diagnosis.

The iridologist looks at the iris through a magnifying glass, photographs it for later study, and on the basis of these observations alone, proceeds to assess your "constitution," health status, and vulnerability to disease. Iridologists claim that the iris contains hundreds of thousands of nerve endings that are connected to every tissue and organ of the body. Any abnormality is said to be reflected in the colors and patterns of the iris, its structure, and degrees of lightness and darkness. Whereas the traditional doctor looks *into* the eyes, the iridologist looks at the iris as if it were a television screen reflecting what's coming *out of* the body.

Iridology was the brainchild of a Hungarian doctor, Ignatz Von Peczely. As the story goes, when Von Peczely was twelve years old, he was walking through a thicket in a forest. The foliage and trees were very dense, shutting out most of the light and leaving his path in semidarkness. While making his way amid the brush and trees, he became aware of two large, yellow eyes staring at him. He was terrified. Suddenly, he found himself being attacked, his arm held in a ferocious grip by what turned out to be a large owl, to whose nest he had inadvertently come too close. Von Peczely was unable to shake his arm loose, and in self-defense he broke the bird's leg. As he did this, he noticed a black line appear in the bird's eyes. He carried the owl home, and after he had nursed it back to health, he noticed that the black line had turned white. The memory of that change remained with him over the years. After he became a physician (and a naturopath), he often noticed similar changes in the irises of his patients, and he became convinced that there was a reflex relationship between the interior organs of the body and the colored portion of the eye. He documented this relationship with complicated charts that are still used in the practice of iridology, although they have been modified over the years. You might say, then, that the founding father of iridology was a frightened twelve-year-old boy. Today, iridology is used throughout the world by herbalists, naturopaths, homeopaths, and other practitioners of alternative medicine.

Perhaps the best-known contemporary iridologist is Bernard Jensen, a doctor who has updated the iris chart that maps the connections from the body to the eye. This chart is superimposed over the image of the iris and its three major and three minor "zones" to identify and interpret any abnormalities. (Other iridologists claim that there are as many as 100 such zones.) Iridologists do not claim to be able to diagnose specific diseases; rather, they say they can identify underlying toxicity and inflammation in the connective tissue of the body, which leave the person vulnerable to both physical and emotional disorders. On the basis of these findings, an iridologist can go on to recommend certain herbs and other "natural" foods to prevent disease. If, after such intervention, a person remains healthy, the credit belongs to the iridologist. According to critics of iridology, that's tantamount to "curing" nonexistent disease.

Let me say, up front, that *none*—not a single one—of the claims made by iridologists has ever been scientifically substantiated. In a large study reported by the University of San Diego in 1979, 143 patients with kidney disease were tested by iridology to see whether it could diagnose their condition. The accuracy of iridology turned out to be no greater than if the practitioners had guessed or flipped a coin. In another series of 762 cases, there was also no correlation whatsoever between iridology and the actual diagnosis. In a third study, 88 percent of healthy persons were incorrectly diagnosed by iridologists as having kidney disease. Presumably, an iridologist would reply, "Maybe not now, but just you wait and see!"

❖ ❖ ❖   The bottom line? Iridology does not appear to have any scientific basis, and none of its findings or claims has ever been reproduced.

❖ 23 ❖

JUICING

What's Better for You,
a Squeeze or a Bite?

Remember when going to the bar meant that you were either a lawyer or looking for a beer or whiskey? These days, however, more and more of us go to alcohol-free bars—and health food stores—to have some freshly squeezed vegetable juice or fruit juice. We do this because, in addition to being delicious, refreshing, and healthful, juice is a convenient way to get the ingredients in fruits and vegetables everyone should have. But is drinking them in their *liquid* form any better for you than eating them solid and raw? That's what we'll be considering in this chapter.

Statistics confirm that fruit and vegetables help prevent cancer and heart disease, probably by strengthening the immune system. Populations with the highest consumption of these foods have the lowest incidence of cancer. The "phytochemicals" they contain—minerals, vitamins, essential fatty acids, carbohydrates, enzymes and other proteins, and countless other substances—act together in their natural state to prevent a variety of diseases. However, taking any of them from a bottle, singly or in combination, is not nearly as effective as eating the natural food or drinking its fresh juice. This was dramatically demonstrated in the case of beta carotene, one of some thirty carotenoids present in fruits and vegetables. We used to think it was the beta carotene, with its antioxidant properties, that protected against heart disease and cancer. Many doctors (including me) used to recommend beta carotene supplements to patients at high risk of malignancy (especially lung cancer) and blood vessel disease. Then came study after study showing that these supplements have no preventive properties. The most convincing research involved almost 1,200 men and women, of whom half were given fifty milligrams of beta carotene daily for more than four years, while the other half received a placebo. Both groups were followed for an additional eight years, at the end of which the results were tabulated. There was no reduction in the incidence of cancer or heart disease among those who had been taking the beta carotene supplements. Other studies have suggested that supplemental beta carotene may even be associated with an *increase* in the rate of deaths from cancer. While it's possible that a longer follow-up period might have revealed some protective effect of carotene, it's more likely that the observed benefits of fruit and vegetables are due to compounds other than beta carotene, or to beta carotene combined with other naturally occurring substances.

Nutritionists and doctors have been squeezing the life (and juice) out of fruits and vegetables for centuries. The popularity of juicing has increased in recent years, largely owing to the salesmanship of Jay Korditch, television's Juiceman. In addition to selling millions of dollars' worth of his own juice extractors (*Consumer Reports* thinks they're over-priced and that units costing considerably less are just as good), Korditch increased public awareness of the hazards of animal fat and the benefits of raw fruits and vegetables. However, he also claimed, or at least implied in his infomercials, that consuming them as fresh juice has unique and important biological advantages. I have, without success, scoured the scientific literature looking for evidence that juicing is better for you, or more effectively satisfies your nutritional requirements, than eating the raw stuff. In my opinion, it makes no difference how you consume your daily quota of these foods, as long as you *do* consume it. There's no reason, as far as I can determine, to juice your fruit and vegetables rather than eat them whole, and preferably raw and fresh. Virtually all the "medical" claims for the superiority of juicing appear to come from "interested parties."

I love fresh fruit juice; I also like some of the vegetable juices, though I personally don't find them as tasty as fruit juice. There is no question that both are good for you. Juices can also be convenient. For example, one pint of fresh vegetable juice is nutritionally equivalent to two large salads; if you prefer to have your salad in liquid form, that's fine. Again, most people would rather drink six or eight ounces of carrot juice than sit around eating a pound of carrots. Both provide the same amount of vitamins B, C, D, E, and K; carotenoids; calcium; phosphorus; potassium; sodium; and a little protein. If you prefer the convenience of juices, drink them. But, as noted above, don't expect any additional, miraculous benefits from them.

There is a *downside* to juices. Drinking fresh juice at a juice bar is one thing; preparing it yourself takes time, is messy, and is likely to be more expensive than eating the fruit and vegetables themselves, or even buying bottled juice off the shelf. For example, squeezing your own orange juice may end up costing you about 30 percent more; preparing your own fresh tomato juice is even more expensive. That's because juicing uses much more of the fresh food. One orange, or half a grapefruit, yields less than a full glass of juice (though it also has fewer calories).

Another inconvenience of home juicing is the time constraint. If you want to do it "by the book," the juice experts say you must juice on schedule, and drink the juice almost immediately. Storing it, even in a refrigerator, causes it to oxidize within minutes and lose some of its potency.

There's also the cost of the juicer, which will run you anywhere from $100 to $2,000. (The Juiceman costs about $300, give or take a few bucks.)

The major disadvantage to obtaining your fruit and vegetable in juice form is that you deprive yourself of the roughage needed for proper digestion. So if you're really into a juice program, make sure to eat at least two servings daily—and preferably more—of fiber-rich food such as whole grains, raw vegetables, and fruits.

Finally, it's worth noting that some people who tolerate whole citrus fruits find juice irritating to the throat and stomach.

Among the *advantages* claimed for juicing is that it breaks down the fiber in fruits and vegetables, allowing you to absorb some ingredients that are otherwise excreted. (Many people, including me, think it's better to leave the fiber intact, so that it can move down the bowel and keep the stool moist to prevent constipation, rather than to absorb its breakdown products.) Another claim made by the proponents of juicing is that juice requires less energy to be digested. I am not aware of any reports in the scientific literature to support this notion.

Juice is also touted for another purpose—fasting. As I indicated in chapter 16, I know of no scientific documentation that fasting, in itself, has any therapeutic value. But if you're going to fast, juice is better than water because it provides some nutrients to keep you going.

A distinct advantage of juicing is that it lets you include a wider variety of fruits and vegetables in your diet than you might normally have. This not only offers new taste opportunities but also provides a wider variety of natural ingredients. For example, the usual fare in most homes includes such staples as apples, oranges, bananas, carrots, celery, lemons, limes, and asparagus. But you can toss more exotic foods into the juicer—mangos, papaya, kale, beetroot, and wheatgrass—and drink them in one fell swoop.

Here are the ingredients of some of the *fruits* that make for tasty drinks:

- *Peaches* have a mild laxative action and are especially rich in potassium.
- *Papaya* contains papain, which has active antiulcer properties. It's also full of potassium and magnesium, both of which are lost in the urine when a person is taking a diuretic ("water pill").
- *Cranberries* are the best natural substance for treating and preventing recurrent urinary tract infections. Cranberry juice prevents bacteria from holding on to the walls of the urinary ducts, and so they are more easily passed out of the urinary system. (*Blueberries* also reduce the incidence of urinary infection.)
- *Pineapple* is rich in iodine (good for thyroid function) and also contains bromelain, which has been found in some experiments to alleviate arthritic pain. For example, in one European study, an orthopedist treated fifty-nine patients who had painful, swollen joints with bromelain

for one to three weeks. The treatment was well tolerated, all the subjects in the study stayed with it, and all were found to have less pain, swelling, and tenderness.

- *Apples* are loaded with calcium, sulfur, silicon, magnesium, iron, and potassium, and their pectin is a good source of fiber. Because they contain sorbitol, a sugar with laxative properties, they not only keep the doctor away but also keep you moving.
- *Oranges* are rich in vitamin C, potassium, and a host of other vitamins and minerals.

The yield and potential benefits from combinations of various *vegetables* are even greater:

- *Carrots* are a treasure-house of natural resources. You name it, they have it, in varying amounts—magnesium, iodine, fluorine, potassium, an abundance of the cancer-fighting carotenoids, and a host of vitamins. And you thought carrots only improved night vision?
- *Beets* (in addition to scaring the wits out of the unsuspecting consumer who sees "blood" in the stool and urine after eating them) are very rich in iron and potassium—great for iron-deficiency anemia. Beet juice also adds a nice color and flavor to other juices and mixes very well with them.
- *Garlic* contains the active ingredient allicin, which lowers cholesterol and blood pressure and, according to some researchers, stimulates the immune system.
- *Parsley* is probably the best breath cleanser and purifier there is. Other claims have also been made for it, ranging from enhancing kidney function to improving eyesight, but its effect on breath is the only action which is documented to my satisfaction and to which I can attest personally.

- *Spinach.* Forget about Popeye's preoccupation with spinach. Although it contains plenty of iron, it's not sufficiently absorbed from the stomach to have given Popeye those great muscles. But this vegetable is abundant in oxalic acid (which relieves constipation but causes kidney stones), vitamin C, calcium, and potassium.

How much fruit and vegetable juice should you drink every day? I recommend at least five servings. What constitutes a serving depends on which fruit or vegetable you choose to squeeze. For example, each of the following is one serving:

- One cup of orange or carrot juice
- One whole apple, pear, or mango
- Half a banana, cantaloupe, or grapefruit
- One cup of uncooked vegetables, or one-half cup cooked

If you decide to go the juice route, you're better off squeezing it yourself. It's more expensive and time-consuming, but you can drink it really fresh—from fruits and vegetables you have bought yourself, and to whose high quality you can attest. When someone else does the buying and squeezing, you never know for sure what you're getting.

Here are some practical tips for the prospective juicer:

- Wash all fruit and vegetables thoroughly before juicing, to get rid of any pesticides, waxes, fertilizer, and other contaminants.
- Remove the rind from oranges, grapefruits, kiwi, and papaya; they contain potentially toxic substances. However, the skins of lemons and limes may safely be included.
- Leave the white pulp of the orange, with its vitamin-rich pectin.

- Cut away the core of the apple: the seeds contain cyanide. However, you may include virtually all other seeds, such as those from lemons, oranges, limes, grapefruit, grapes, and melons.
- Do not juice celery leaves. They're bitter and can ruin the taste of the celery juice.
- When shopping for carrots, buy the larger ("horse") ones. They're easier to peel, and because they're usually too big to be sold in a bag, you can pick and choose the best ones individually.
- Consult your health food store about what juicer to buy. Most people are familiar with the type used to make orange or lemon juice. A hydraulic press extractor, though considerably more expensive, retains more of the minerals than the other types. It will even juice peanuts, watermelon (with rind), grapes, and many other foods.
- Very sweet juice (from pears, grapes, beets, apples, or carrots) that you've made yourself should *not* be drunk "straight" or undiluted. Mix it with equal parts of water, or with another juice that's not as sweet. Undiluted, it's cloying, it's more difficult to digest, and it may cause gas and bloating. Also, the sudden concentrated sugar load may be too much for diabetics and people with hypoglycemia.
- For some reason, juice mavens advise preparing and drinking fruits and vegetables separately, several hours apart. They say that improves digestion and assimilation and produces much less gas. They also suggest drinking the fruit juice in the morning and the vegetable juice in the evening. I have discussed these recommendations with dietitians, nutritionists, and other doctors and have been unable to confirm their importance, wisdom, or necessity. The carbohydrate load in each is very similar, and there is no obvious reason to take them separately.

- You may prefer to filter the vegetable juice, to remove the grit it often contains.
- Avoid any fruit or vegetable to which you are allergic. Juicing it won't eliminate the allergy.

The Juiceman himself is now promoting *capsules* as an equivalent alternative to fresh juice and maintains that they contain essentially the same ingredients. His product is made by a technique called low-temperature spray-drying, which extracts the water in the fruits and vegetables; the residual powder is then put into capsules. (There are several whole-juice capsules now on the market, each with its own technology—"Easy Juicing" and "Juice Plus" are among those I have tried. One month's supply of both the fruits and the vegetables costs about $50.) There have been several reports, virtually all sponsored by the manufacturers, that claim that these capsules are the nutritional equivalent of the fruits and vegetables from which they are derived.

❖ ❖ ❖   What's the bottom line? Juicing is largely a matter of personal preference, and an acceptable way of getting the fruits and vegetables you need—fun for some, but inconvenient for others. It's particularly useful for persons who can't bite or chew food. It can be messy, and it is sometimes more expensive than eating the whole fruits and vegetables. If you only drink their juice, supplement your diet with high-fiber foods to make up for fiber lost in the juicing process. Capsules containing dehydrated fresh fruits and vegetables are probably acceptable alternatives to juicing.

❖ 24 ❖

LIGHT THERAPY

Let There Be Light!

Millions of people are happy, contented, and calm all through the spring and summer months. But when the days become shorter, and darkness envelops them, they become sad, irritable, depressed, and moody; they have insomnia; they either lose their appetite or gorge themselves on pasta and ice cream. During those dark winter months, they're a mess. Then comes the spring, and they begin to perk up. By the time summer rolls around again, most of them are back to their old selves—until the fall restarts the downward spiral. Some people who have borderline depression year-round manage to cope during the summer months, but their condition worsens dramatically when winter sets in.

That this behavior is clearly related to exposure to light was not appreciated by scientific medicine until quite recently, but the alternative folks have known about it for centuries. The Ayurvedic doctor Deepak Chopra points out that the Hippocrates of the Ayurvedic community, a physician named Charaka who lived in the sixth century B.C., recommended sunlight to treat a variety of diseases, presumably including the depression of darkness—appropriately referred to as SAD (seasonal affective disorder). Not until the 1970s did Western scientists come to realize that these debilitating symptoms were in some way associated with light deprivation. This theory is now widely accepted, even though it remains unclear how absence of light produces these symptoms, or how adding light to the environment corrects them. (According to one theory, light suppresses the overproduction of melatonin, an excess of which may cause depression and fatigue.)

The human body has several rhythms, all controlled by the flow and production of various hormones and other chemicals. The menstrual cycle, hunger signals, and patterns of waking and sleeping have their own rhythms. Waking and sleeping are dependent on light rays striking the retina, whose receptors transmit these impulses to various parts of the brain. They "inform" the brain that daylight has arrived, that it's time to wake up and get going, or that it's time to sleep. These signals are our built-in alarm clock. When they are not forthcoming, as occurs when the days are short, the brain and the body presumably function at the same low level of energy as when you are asleep. That may be an oversimplification, but it makes the point. The logical conclusion from all this is that people who develop the SAD syndrome should be treated by increased exposure to light. And that's exactly what's being done, with excellent results.

Light is such a powerful "wake-up" stimulant that an older man whose enlarged prostate makes it necessary for him to empty his bladder frequently during the night may quite seriously be cautioned to do so in the dark. Turning the lights on so that he can see what he's doing may wake him up—at two A.M. and keep him awake! Another recent study shows that if you read for any length of time before going to sleep, the exposure even to that relatively low concentration of light can contribute to insomnia. This suggests that while considerable light—10,000 lux—is needed to treat SAD, much less intense sources, even candlelight, can also have a beneficial effect. (I don't understand the figure 10,000 lux any better than you do. It apparently has something to do with candlepower, which lighting companies can explain to you when you order lamps from them.)

When doctors first realized the importance of light in the treatment of SAD, all manner of therapeutic light products appeared on the market. These fancy light boxes were expensive and, as it turned out, unnecessary. Recent research has shown that all you need is a high-intensity fluorescent lamp that delivers 10,000-lux illumination (make sure it's the kind that screens out harmful ultraviolet light). If you have been diagnosed with SAD, you will improve within days after sitting under one of these lamps for fifteen minutes to three hours daily, preferably in the early morning or at dusk. Don't look directly into the light; that can hurt your eyes. Sit under the lamp where the light falls on the book or paper you're reading.

Despite the therapeutic effect of light, you should continue your antidepressant prescription if you have a year-round problem that is worsened when winter comes.

❖ 25 ❖

MAGNETIC THERAPY
Are You Positive or Negative?

Over the years, scientists, pseudoscientists, and interested laypersons have been fascinated by the idea that magnetic energy may cause disease—and may also cure it. This interest spawned a number of fads, one of which I remember from my childhood. My father used to sit for hours in a big metal box whose mysterious magnetic emanations were supposed to cure whatever ailed him. It was the invention of our family doctor—a medical Rube Goldberg and a frustrated Alexander Graham Bell. And you know what? Dad left that box every evening feeling better than he had felt all day!

Modern consumer interest in magnetic fields has most recently been focused on the antennas of cellular phones. (You should not use a cellular phone if you have a pacemaker, because the phone discombobulates its function. Hospitals do not permit you to use such a phone near anyone with a pacemaker.) Many other electronic devices also create magnetic fields, which make them suspect in the minds of many people. Here are some examples:

- Microwave ovens (one of my sons still won't have one in his kitchen, because he's "sure" that the electromagnetic energy it emits causes cancer)
- Power stations (living near a power station seems to be associated with an increased risk of leukemia)
- Television sets and computer screens (perhaps parents use the fact that they generate energy fields as an excuse for limiting their kids' TV viewing—"Turn the TV off, David dear, or you'll be zapped, turn green, and glow in the dark")
- Fluorescent lighting (often hard to avoid, especially on the job)
- Electrical wiring at home and at work (to which there's no alternative)
- Hair dryers (which my wife insists on using)
- Electric razors (another one of my sons has given his up— he doesn't believe the close shave is worth the risk)
- Electric blankets (which have been rightly or wrongly blamed for the greater incidence of miscarriages these days)

Despite the fear of exposure to the magnetic energy that surrounds us, there has been little, if any, confirmation that any of the sources listed above can really make us sick. Still, where there's smoke . . .

The body's various energy processes generate their own magnetic fields, which modern technological advances now enable us to demonstrate and measure. For example, the human brain emits electrical currents of two cycles per second while we're asleep, and as many as twenty cycles per second when we're awake. (The current in most American homes is sixty cycles per second.) We are now enhancing and using these fields in several ways. Here are just two examples: MRI (magnetic resonance imaging), a major diagnostic tool, works because it interprets our bodies' magnetic energy. This same energy field is also what makes magnets applied to a fractured limb speed the healing process.

Some enthusiasts claim that manipulation of the body's magnetic fields has vast untapped therapeutic potential. Wolfgang Ludwig, director of the Institute for Biophysics in Horb, Germany, recently wrote, "Magnetic field therapy is a method that penetrates the whole human body and can treat every organ without chemical side effects." He believes that magnetic therapy can treat many disorders from stress to cancer, from blood vessel disease to infections. Several references, particularly in mainstream Eastern European and Russian medical journals, support his conclusions, although few successful studies of magnetic therapy have been documented in the Western literature. I suspect that many of those metal boxes like the one my father sat in some sixty years ago (or similar contraptions) are still being peddled.

I had not been convinced that magnetic therapy is useful for anything beyond accelerating the healing of fractured bones. Then, some years ago, I met Robert Holcomb, a distinguished neurologist at Vanderbilt University, in Nashville. While researching new techniques for controlling chronic pain, he observed that placing small magnets on selected parts of the body often reduces or eliminates pain due to a variety of causes. He showed me, under his electron microscope, how these magnets alter the orientation of the chromosomes within cells. He is convinced that this shift in position of the chromosomes leads to relief of acute and chronic pain.

Four years ago, at my suggestion, one of my relatives with a chronic back problem went to see Holcomb. After determining that her pain was due to severe muscle spasm, he placed several magnets on carefully selected sites of her body (correct positioning is crucial). She noticed some improvement within hours; after she'd been wearing the magnets for one week, and without any additional physiotherapy or massage, most of her pain had disappeared. Now, four years later, she still applies her magnets several times a week, and she credits them for her continued improvement.

However, other patients whom I've referred to Holcomb have not responded nearly as well, or not at all. I have no idea why some do and others don't, or what role the placebo effect (see chapter 2) plays in these cases. But I have a gut feeling (admittedly anecdotal and unscientific) that there may be something to the magnet theory and magnetic therapy. It's probably because looking at those cells under electron microscopy impressed me, although I don't pretend to understand how realigning chromosomes lessens pain.

Several magnetotherapy pain clinics have sprung up around the country, some of which are using Holcomb's method. They may be worth looking into, if you have a chronic pain problem.

❖ ❖ ❖   What's the bottom line? The one specific, proven therapeutic effect of magnetotherapy is its acceleration of the healing of bone fractures. However, there is growing interest in and experience with this approach for pain control. If you suffer from chronic pain, magnetotherapy is worth looking into. You might telephone Robert Holcomb's clinic (615-329-9629) for further information.

❖ 26 ❖

MIND-BODY THERAPY

It's "All in Your Head"?
Don't You Believe It!

When I was a medical student, the curriculum dealt only with "real" diseases. My teachers had the time and patience only for symptoms that could be seen (a rash), heard (a murmur), felt (a lump), smelled (the characteristic odor associated with certain diseases), or documented in an *objective* test (blood or urine test, X ray, electrocardiogram). Complaints with no measurable physiological basis were deemed "all in the head"; these patients weren't "really sick," and we referred them directly to a psychiatrist.

Times have changed. Today, most doctors and patients (not to mention medical school professors and their students) are convinced of the link between physical disorders and emotional stress. We appreciate, for example, that serious disease can depress you, and that chronic depression can make you seriously ill.

We don't need a double-blind, placebo-controlled study to know that people can "die of fright"—that when we're scared, the heart pounds, the blood pressure rises, the mouth becomes dry, and we may lose control of the bowel or bladder, or break out in a cold sweat. When you're embarrassed or angry, doesn't your face become flushed, blotchy, or red—very much like what happens during an allergic reaction? Put all these observations together, and you've made a case for the unity of mind and body. It's amazing that it took so long for us to figure this out. For the truth is that symptoms resulting from emotional stress are often indistinguishable from symptoms of "organic" disease.

A temporary blush or a transient rise in heart rate, blood pressure, or cholesterol in response to a short-lived emotional crisis may not harm you, but such reactions will do you no good if the stress is ongoing. The classic example is the documented observation in one particular study that men who have lost their wives to cancer have a death rate two to twelve times higher than that of married men of the same age.

The immune system, about which we are learning more all the time, coordinates our mental processes and bodily functions. It controls how effectively we ward off infection, cancer, heart attacks, strokes, and virtually every other illness that can befall us, and even how rapidly we become "old." Many of the chemicals, blood cells, hormones, and other components of the immune system have been identified and can be measured. This has led to the development of *psychoneuroimmunology,* a new and important medical discipline devoted to the understanding and documentation of the mind-body relationship.

Eastern cultures and religions have for thousands of years been aware of this unity and have evolved techniques to influence it. In modern society, this has largely been the domain of practitioners of alternative medicine. I have already described several of these methods—including aromatherapy (see chapter 6), Ayurveda (see chapter 7), and hypnosis (see chapter 21). In this chapter, I examine three others that are widely used: biofeedback, guided imagery, and meditation.

Biofeedback

Biofeedback directs or manipulates physiological responses which we normally allow to proceed at their own pace and which, until recently, we didn't even know we could control. This technique, based on the pioneering work of an experimental psychologist, Neal Miller, in the 1960s, is now widely used by both conventional and alternative practitioners. Unlike several of the "complementary" methods described elsewhere in this book, biofeedback has been thoroughly studied and reported in the scientific literature. Although there are some differences of opinion regarding exactly how effective it is, and in what circumstances, there is a consensus that it can be useful. The results of biofeedback therapy are not always as clear-cut and permanent as, say, surgical removal of an infected appendix, but they can be impressive. I've observed favorable responses to biofeedback among my own patients time and again.

Here's how biofeedback works. The nervous system has two major components—voluntary and involuntary, or autonomic. The voluntary component is totally under your control. If you want to move your leg or arm, you simply decide to do it, and your brain does the rest. It sends a message to the appropriate muscle groups, and *voilà,* the leg moves. You want to dance; you dance. You want to raise a cup of coffee to your lips; your wish is your brain's command. By contrast, the autonomic nervous system goes its merry way without any input from you. Take respiration, for example. You can speed up or slow down the rate at which you breathe, but try holding your breath indefinitely—your autonomic nervous system won't let you do it. This system makes it possible to go through life virtually unaware of your breathing except when you've been exerting yourself, or if you have an underlying heart or lung problem. The same is true of such other bodily functions as heart rate, blood pressure, and skin temperature. However, a biofeedback therapist can teach you how to control many inner mechanisms, not only voluntary and but also autonomic, including muscle tension, heart rate, blood supply to the skin, and even your emotions.

Here's how it's done. First, the biofeedback therapist attaches monitoring electrodes to your body; their location depends on what physiologic process is being monitored. If it's your heart rate, blood pressure, muscle tension, or skin temperature, they're applied to the skin. If the purpose of the biofeedback is to treat mood disorders, attention deficit disorder and hyperactivity, spasms associated with cerebral palsy, seizures, sleep problems, headache, or grinding of the teeth at night, the electrodes will be attached to your scalp in order to obtain an electroencephalogram (EEG), which monitors brain waves. The electrodes are connected to a computer, a polygraph, or another instrument that emits a signal indicating the intensity or level of the process to be controlled.

Next, as you lie there, you'll be told to listen to tones or watch the display on a meter or computer screen. What you hear or see reflects the intensity of the underlying bodily process on which you're focusing.

Then, you'll concentrate on trying to influence the process by performing specific mental exercises in which you consciously visualize certain images that affect your mood. After eight to ten sessions, most people can usually relax specific muscles, raise or lower heart rate, decrease blood pressure, break a bronchial spasm, control intestinal function, or alter any of several other automatic functions.

The greatest reward of successful self-regulation is relaxation and reduction of stress. Many other health benefits derive from this. Physical symptoms that have been credibly shown to respond to biofeedback include Raynaud's syndrome or disease (in which small blood vessels go into painful spasm); asthma; high blood pressure; epilepsy; attention deficit disorder and hyperactivity; migraine and tension headaches; chronic insomnia; fecal and urinary incontinence (a serious problem among the elderly, diabetics, and patients with inflammatory bowel disease, spinal cord injuries, or postsurgical difficulties); chronic constipation (especially in children); irritable bowel syndrome; motion sickness; various neuromuscular disorders; the pain of arthritis and muscle spasm; anxiety; and depression.

In attempting to document biofeedback's track record, I decided to survey at random twelve reports from the world literature. I limited this initial search to the area of rehabilitation medicine, in order to determine the effect of combining biofeedback with traditional measures in the treatment of subjects with disabling injuries. Among these twelve studies, two reported definite improvement, one concluded with a "maybe," six failed to show any impact, and three found that biofeedback alone was no more effective than conventional methods. However, when I looked at the data in the management of Raynaud's disease, high blood pressure, and tension headaches, results with biofeedback were more impressive. In sum, it appears that biofeedback has varying outcomes—there are some hits, some runs, and a few strikeouts.

If your doctor believes in the potential of biofeedback, he or she can refer you to one of the more than 10,000 biofeedback professionals in the United States, at least 2,000 of whom are nationally certified.

❖ ❖ ❖ The bottom line? Biofeedback is a legitimate technique that can be useful in a wide variety of conditions. It is more effective for some disorders than others, but is worth a try under any circumstances because it is noninvasive, generally cost-effective, and harmless.

Guided Imagery

Guided imagery is a mind-body technique that lies somewhere between hypnosis and biofeedback; it relies very heavily on the power of suggestion. It has been credited, at least anecdotally, with lessening anxiety, improving mood, and controlling or easing pain. None of these claims surprises me, but I have trouble believing that guided imagery can cause a tumor to disappear, as has been reported but never documented.

Unlike biofeedback, guided imagery requires no instruments to monitor your response. The therapist asks you to conjure up a specific image on which you focus intently enough to convince your subconscious that it is real. Of course, such imaging happens all the time when we daydream or fantasize. Two examples that come to mind are a "spontaneous" erection induced by a sexually stimulating thought and a racing heart in anticipation of something exciting or threatening. Now, imagine that you're cutting into a ripe lemon, squeezing some of the juice, and tasting it. Don't you feel that characteristic tingling sensation in your salivary glands? If you do, you've just experienced a successful mini-session in guided imagery.

Some of the accounts of the use of guided imagery are fascinating. For example, one woman with severe pain in her hip was asked to describe her symptoms in detail. She said she felt as if someone were plunging a knife into the area and turning it. The therapist then had her imagine that she was grasping and slowly removing it. As she did so, her pain virtually disappeared. Many people with cancer are asked to visualize, as realistically as possible, a mass of cancerous tissue being attacked by cells from the immune system. I have seen no documented reports of cures or remissions following such sessions, but I can understand how they would help restore a patient's sense of control in the face of life-threatening illness. In fact, improving the patients' outlook and having them involved in their own health care are the strongest arguments in favor of guided imagery.

This approach is being incorporated in several conventional hospitals. One in particular, Marin General Hospital in the San Francisco Bay Area, has established a guided imagery service under the direction of a psychologist trained in holistic health care and conducted by a trained staff. It is free for inpatients and is also available to the public for a fee, which is reimbursed by some third-party payers. Each session lasts just under an hour. The initial goal is total relaxation. Participants learn breathing techniques to help them achieve the inner calm necessary for imagery to be successful. Once they are completely relaxed, they then focus on where it hurts (the program is mainly for cancer patients) and try to modify their pain by imagining a pleasurable scene or situation—the site of a great vacation, or a beautiful mountain, beach, or garden. In other cases, they conjure up a wise person or an inner guide whom they can ask for solutions to the problem at hand. Marin General Hospital is claiming that guided imagery does help its patients cope with their stress and pain.

❖ ❖ ❖   What's the bottom line? If you are being treated for a chronic problem that has left you stressed and worried, try adding guided imagery to the treatment. It may make you feel better, but don't expect it to cure the underlying condition.

Meditation

Meditation is similar to but less structured than biofeedback and guided imagery. It's also easier to do on your own without the help of a therapist. Like the other techniques, it can be used to reduce stress.

Calming and focusing the mind, which is basically what meditation is all about, is very old hat. The most abundant literature on the subject originates in Eastern religions—Chinese, Japanese, and Indian. Although we think of meditation as something private, quiet, and sedentary, there are forms that involve other people or movement. These include the Chinese and Japanese martial arts (such as tai chi and aikido, respectively), the walking of Zen Buddhism, and the yoga component of Ayurveda.

In the 1960s, the Maharishi Mahesh Yogi came to the United States from India for the purpose of introducing transcendental meditation (TM) in a form more acceptable to Western tastes. This new version is much less demanding than the homegrown product, and TM has indeed caught on. Its popularity has been greatly increased by the endorsement and support of Deepak Chopra, one of the Maharishi's pupils and now a luminary in his own right. There are TM centers throughout the country, there is a Maharishi International University in Indiana (not India), and TM is currently big, big business.

One of the greatest factors in the acceptance of TM has been the interest and involvement of Herbert Benson of Harvard, who coined the term "relaxation response" for his own particular application of TM. For the past twenty-five years, Benson has been conducting studies of meditation that have yielded impressive and believable results. His findings, as well as those of other investigators, were recently summarized in a report to the Office on Alternative Medical Systems and Practices of the National Institutes of Health. Here are some of the more important conclusions:

- Meditation reduces blood levels of cortisol, the stress hormone.
- Meditation is associated with a longer life span, better quality of life, fewer hospitalizations, and reduced health care costs.
- Regular meditation allays anxiety and reduces the severity of chronic pain.
- Blood pressure (and heart rate) can be lowered by meditation, especially in African-Americans. I have seen this in a minority (no pun intended) of my own patients with moderately elevated but not very high blood pressure. "Lowered," here, does not mean "normalized," but such patients often need less medication.
- Meditation can decrease blood cholesterol. (Stress, we know, can raise it, so it's entirely reasonable that reducing stress can have the opposite effect.)
- Meditation is a useful adjunct in controlling substance abuse.

I learned long ago that in medicine, as in politics, there is no such thing as unanimity. Despite the rave reviews from the millions of people who practice meditation, it apparently has a potential downside. A relatively small number who try it develop negative feelings about themselves and may even become disoriented; some schizophrenics were reported to have become acutely psychotic after meditating. Although it's important to be aware of these complications, they should not diminish your ardor for the process if you feel better doing it.

There are several different ways to meditate, and everyone develops his or her own preferences. (My wife is so adept at meditating that she can do it while riding in a car—as a passenger, of course.) Although you can learn to meditate from any number of books and manuals, I think you're better off getting initial instruction from an expert. Virtually any holistically oriented doctor or psychologist can teach you. Here's one way to do it.

- Twice every day, preferably before breakfast and dinner, choose a quiet place and sit in a comfortable chair with both feet on the ground (don't lie down).
- Breathe easily and naturally, preferably (but not necessarily) with your eyes closed. Ease into this relaxed state for about a minute.
- Now it's "mantra" time. A mantra is a phrase or word that you repeat to yourself (not out loud); it distracts you from other thoughts. "Om" is a very popular mantra among people who practice TM, but a mantra could be "two," or "love," or any sound that pleases you. Concentrate on your breathing as you think of your mantra.
- Don't resist any thoughts that come to mind. Accept them—roll with the punches, so to speak—and return to your mantra. As you continue to inhale and exhale quietly, thinking the mantra, these thoughts will gradually fade away. You may or may not "feel" relaxed at this point, but it doesn't matter. Believe me, you soon will be relaxed.
- Spend about fifteen or twenty minutes just thinking of the mantra and breathing softly and regularly. When you're through, stand up slowly and gradually return to the swing of things.

Devote twenty minutes twice a day to this kind of simple meditation. Let all the thoughts and plans that constantly ferment in your mind drift away. View meditation as a mental cleansing, an opportunity to become aware of your inner self. Statistics aside, it's good for you. Let the epidemiologists worry whether or not it prevents disease; leave it to the government bureaucrats to decide whether it reduces the costs of health care. That's not your major concern; feeling better is. And don't worry if you fall asleep. If you do, it won't detract from the value of the process, as long as you don't use meditation as a sleeping aid.

There are many different ways to optimize the mind-body relationship. Stress can be reduced by praying (some "non-believers" say that prayer is simply a longer mantra), art therapy, music therapy, therapeutic touching, and on and on. Try whatever works for you. Entire books have been written on the mind-body relationship and how to modify or influence it. The field is complex and fascinating. If you want to know more about some of what I have touched upon, read *Mind/Body Medicine,* edited by Daniel Goldman and Joel Gurin (Consumer Reports Books, 1993).

❖ ❖ ❖   The bottom line? There is objective evidence that meditation can reduce blood pressure, heart rate, and the concentration of stress hormones (cortisol) in the bloodstream. But that's not the only reason to meditate. Everyone I know who meditates correctly and regularly enjoys it and feels better.

❖ 27 ❖

NEUROLINGUISTIC PROGRAMMING (NLP)

Watch Your Language!

Neurolinguistic programming (NLP) isn't easy to understand in any of its descriptions, at least not those that I reviewed. I can best explain it as a mind-body technique that combines psychotherapy and imaging. The basic premise is that the words we use reflect an inner, subconscious perception of our problems; if these words and perceptions are inaccurate, as long as we continue to use and to think them, our underlying problem will persist. In other words, our attitudes are, in a sense, a self-fulfilling prophecy. The neurolinguistic therapist analyzes every word and phrase you use when you describe your symptoms or concerns about your health, watching your facial expressions and body movements as you express them. He or she then helps you remodel your thoughts and mental associations in order to fix your preconceived notions.

The goal of NLP is to get you to change your view of your emotional or physical problem. Therapy then goes on to replace negative perceptions with positive ones by means of skillful imaging (see chapter 26). It seems to me that NLP operates much like increased suggestibility in hypnosis (see chapter 21), although this is vigorously denied by NLP practitioners. For example, David Paul, the medical director of the Vail Medical Center, who no doubt is called upon to treat many skiing injuries in that neck of the woods, describes how he is able to manipulate a displaced shoulder back into its socket by positive commands such as "allow your arm to relax," and "the discomfort is more bearable," and so on. It's apparent that this form of mind-body medicine, essentially a form of psychotherapy, can be used to treat virtually any problem—from cancer to phobia. However, I am not aware of any scientific documentation for its success.

You can learn more about NLP by writing to the Dynamic Learning Center (P. O. Box 1112, Ben Lomond, CA 95005; telephone 408-336-3457). The center will provide you with additional reading material and the names of practitioners near where you live. It's probably not an unbiased source, but it's as reliable as any.

OXYGEN THERAPY
Good Health—Out of Thin Air?

You can't survive without oxygen. When an artery that supplies one of your vital organs, such as the heart or brain, suddenly becomes blocked and can no longer deliver oxygen-bearing blood, you'll have a heart attack or stroke; you might even die. However, even if you don't have a diseased artery, you can still be oxygen-deprived. If you're mountain climbing at a very high altitude, or if the oxygen-delivery system in the cabin of your airplane suddenly breaks down at 30,000 feet, your tissues will get precious little oxygen even though your arteries are wide open.

Everyone agrees that supplemental oxygen is good for you when there's not enough oxygen available, but some practitioners of alternative medicine believe that everyone should have a little (or a lot) more—especially (but not only) people with underlying health problems. In the opinion of these practitioners, the vital role of oxygen in human health and disease is not fully appreciated. And that's what the dispute between conventional and complementary medicine is all about.

Why such a fuss about having more oxygen than nature and the environment normally provide? The problem, believe it or not, is that like so many things in life (with the possible exception of knowledge, sex, and money), more oxygen is *not* always better. In fact, it can actually harm you. Here's an example. Doctors used to think that every premature infant should be given supplemental oxygen. Perfectly reasonable, right? After all, these babies are tiny and fragile, and their lungs may not be sufficiently developed to oxygenate their blood. So for years, all preemies received extra oxygen. But then it was noted that those who survived developed visual problems due to clouding of the lens of the eye (retrolental fibroplasia). The extra oxygen they were given at birth had stimulated the production of scar tissue in the normally clear lens, leaving it opaque and difficult to see through. There are other potential complications from excess oxygen, described below.

The proponents of "hyperoxygenation" say that while healthy tissues thrive on oxygen, sick, cancerous cells and infectious agents (such as bacteria, viruses, and fungi) decay and die in an oxygen-rich environment. According to them, we should be using oxygen—which is plentiful, readily available, and cheap—as a therapeutic agent instead of focusing on micronutrients and other drugs that really don't work. Are they right? In some cases, yes. There are some legitimate circumstances that call for extra oxygen in one of several forms. (Although oxygen is a gas usually delivered by mask or nasal prongs, it can also be given under pressure, or as ozone, or as a liquid in the form of hydrogen peroxide.)

Hyperbaric Oxygen Therapy

Hyperbaric oxygen therapy has been used for over a hundred years, though more so in Europe than in the United States, where its indications are limited, clear-cut, and well defined. The term "hyperbaric oxygen" refers to the intermittent inhalation of 100 percent pure oxygen delivered for varying periods of time under high pressure—ranging from 2.5 to as many as 6 atmospheres (oxygen pressure at sea level is 1 atmosphere). Such high concentrations, under pressure, can be delivered by special masks or in long, thin, pressurized chambers sealed to provide the desired amount of oxygen. There are several hundred larger, much more expensive hyperbaric chambers available in various centers that can accommodate as many as fourteen patients at a time. Here are some of the conditions for which hyperbaric oxygen is prescribed.

The bends (decompression sickness)

When a deep-sea diver comes up from the depths too quickly, nitrogen gas bubbles enter his or her bloodstream. When these bubbles are large enough to block a major artery, they can be fatal. Hyberbaric oxygen not only shrinks these bubbles so that they do not obstruct the arteries, it also nourishes tissues whose blood supply was cut off. Because hyperbaric oxygen is lifesaving in these circumstances, the Undersea Medical Society in the United States lobbied successfully for the introduction of hyperbaric chambers in this country specifically to treat the bends.

Air embolism

Arteries can be blocked by air bubbles that can form during surgery, or when introduced accidentally into the bloodstream by an intravenous injection, or during dialysis, or when a lung is inadvertently punctured (as, for example, during a biopsy). Here too, hyperbaric oxygen reduces the size of the bubbles and restores the flow of blood so that additional oxygen can reach the affected tissues.

Carbon monoxide poisoning

Colorless, odorless, deadly carbon monoxide is responsible for at least half of all fatal poisonings in the United States. If you've been sitting in your car while it's parked in your garage, with the motor running and the windows shut, I can only assume that either you're trying to end it all or you have a limited IQ. Whatever the reason, the carbon monoxide will kill you. Here, too, the treatment of choice is hyperbaric oxygen, which causes oxygen to displace the lethal carbon monoxide in your blood and tissues.

Crush injuries

When a limb or some other part of the body has been crushed, and its arteries squished, gangrene sets in. Delivering high concentrations of oxygen under pressure can help make the tissues viable again and stimulates regrowth of the damaged blood vessels.

Radiation therapy

When a cancer is treated by radiation, the X rays may destroy blood vessels in the area. Hyperbaric oxygen promotes the formation of new blood vessels and revitalizes damaged tissues. This treatment is not used as often as it should be, because it costs so much. If you are being radiated, and you know of a facility or hospital nearby that has this equipment, discuss with your doctor the feasibility of going there.

Bone infection

It is sometimes difficult to cure a bone that's been infected by organisms invading it from the surrounding tissues (for example, in osteomyelitis). In such cases, in addition to the proper antibiotic, some doctors recommend hyperbaric oxygen to promote the growth of new, healthy bone. This is a reasonable addition to the conventional treatment of osteomyelitis, but unfortunately it is not always available—again because of its cost. It's worth asking for.

Burns

A hyperbaric chamber can also help patients with severe and extensive burns. The increased oxygen promotes and accelerates healing.

These are the universally accepted indications for hyperbaric oxygen. However, it is also used for other purposes, some of which medical doctors believe are either inappropriate or ineffective. Here are some examples of gray areas in which further investigation should be done, as well as conditions in which hyberbaric oxygen is of no value.

AIDS

People with AIDS often experience profound fatigue, as well as numbness, or a sensation of "pins and needles" in their limbs. These symptoms are thought to result from injury to nerve cells by HIV, the virus that causes AIDS. Drugs such as AZT, ddl, and ddC may actually worsen matters; but according to some doctors, hyperbaric oxygen can help. The studies I have reviewed suggest that patients with these complaints usually do feel better after treatment with hyperbaric oxygen, though there is no objective evidence that it has any impact on the overall course of their disease. Since ongoing hyperbaric oxygen is so expensive, and because it is only palliative, not curative, our cost-conscious insurers do not usually recommend or pay for it.

Because their immune system has been damaged by HIV, people with AIDS are sitting ducks for any bug that comes along. Hyperbaric oxygen therapy has been shown to increase their resistance to these "opportunistic" infections. Unfortunately, because the number of people with AIDS is so great, and the availability of hyperbaric chambers is so limited, hyperbaric oxygen therapy is not likely to be a real option for most such patients—at least not in the foreseeable future.

Stroke

European doctors are enthusiastic about hyperbaric oxygen for vascular and arterial problems and claim impressive results with it. The rationale of delivering oxygen to deprived tissues seems entirely reasonable. For example, hyperbaric oxygen is a recognized and approved therapy for stroke in most European countries. Reports from Germany credit this treatment with a 71 percent reduction in the cost of care after a stroke. We do not use it very much for strokes in this country because of its limited availability and its cost. This is an area worth looking into, but in the present climate of therapeutic minimalism, where the emphasis is on reducing costs rather than improving the quality of care, I'm not optimistic that it will be pursued. So, if you are unlucky enough to have a stroke while you're in Europe, don't refuse the oxygen-chamber treatment just because you've never heard of it.

Cancer

There have been claims that hyperbaric oxygen can reduce the toxic symptoms associated with chemotherapy of cancer. That may or may not be so, but in any case, there are simpler, less expensive, and equally effective ways to deal with these symptoms.

Multiple sclerosis

Despite many practitioners' claims, I am not aware of any evidence that hyperbaric oxygen alleviates the symptoms or alters the course of multiple sclerosis. The claims of improvements achieved by hyperbaric oxygen have never been substantiated. Don't waste your time and money on it.

Senility or Alzheimer's disease

Alleviation of these disorders by hyperbaric oxygen has never been substantiated. Forget it.

Oxygen treatment is not without its dangers. Complications can occur both as a result of the elevated pressure at which the oxygen is delivered, and from too much of it. For example, any cavity in the body that normally contains air—such as the lung, stomach, or ear ducts—can be hurt by additional pressure. The most common such complication involves the middle ear. When oxygen is introduced under pressure to a blocked eustachian tube (the duct that leads from the throat to the middle ear), the middle ear can become deformed and its membrane can rupture. In someone with severe emphysema, who has overinflated lungs to begin with, hyperbaric oxygen can cause a lung to collapse (pneumothorax). Oxygen under high pressure can rupture an artery in the lung and cause air embolism; long-term administration of oxygen can also produce cataracts. Despite all these possible complications, the benefits of hyperbaric oxygen, when it's needed, far outweigh these risks.

We now come to the more controversial aspects of oxygen (oxidative) therapy—the use of *ozone* and *hydrogen peroxide*.

Ozone

There is considerable difference of opinion, not to mention hostility and frustration, concerning the usefulness of ozone. Its advocates are convinced that it destroys most strains of bacteria, viruses, and fungi, inhibits the growth of some cancer cells, and slows or halts the course of AIDS. They go so far as to claim that it would eliminate most human illnesses and put the pharmaceutical industry out of business altogether! According to them, ozone is banned in the United States (although it is legally available in sixteen other countries—Brazil, Israel, several European nations, and Australia) because our medical establishment and the FDA have "sold out" to the pharmaceutical industry. The reason? Since ozone is a natural substance and cannot be patented (except for its delivery systems), there's no profit to be made by the drug companies. They'd rather we use the more expensive (and profitable) synthetic products they concoct. But as a longtime practicing physician, and a member of many medical organizations and government advisory councils, I can tell you this: I've never had anyone discuss this or any similar issue with me, canvass me, or even remotely suggest that I exert pressure on any regulatory agency to ban any drug. No doctor I know has ever been party to such a conspiracy either. So I wonder who the "bad guys" are in this scenario, where they have been hiding, and with whom they've been conspiring.

Ozone (O_3), discovered in 1840, is oxygen (O_2) with three atoms instead of two. The extra atom comes on board when oxygen is exposed to ultraviolet light or to a strong electrical field. (Ozone is what gives air its fresh, sweet smell after a summer storm.) When ozone enters the bloodstream, by whatever route, it boosts the oxygen level by giving off that extra atom. It does this quite readily because three atoms are not as stable as two.

What does that extra oxygen atom do for you? Here, according to the proponents of ozone, is a partial list of its claimed benefits:

- Ozone activates enzymes that break down "free radicals," the end products of metabolism widely believed (but never really proved) to increase the risk of cancer, accelerate the aging process, and produce the plaques that narrow our arteries.
- When exposed to ozone, the hemoglobin molecule in the red blood cells releases its oxygen more easily, making a greater amount available to the tissues.
- Ozone alters the internal metabolism of cells, making them more resistant to cancer.
- When exposed to ozone, red blood cells do not clump together as readily and become more pliable, so that they can squeeze more easily through a narrowed opening within the blood vessels. The blood also has less tendency to clot.
- The immune system is stimulated by ozone to produce more white blood cells to fight infection.
- Ozone causes several biochemical reactions within the body that render invading bacteria, viruses, and fungi more susceptible to natural defense mechanisms.

Who needs this extra oxygen provided by ozone? Obviously, anyone who has too little oxygen for whatever reason. But according to the proponents of "hyperoxygenation," "healthy" people are also oxygen-deprived because the air we all breathe is usually polluted. At sea level, oxygen should constitute 20 percent of the atmosphere. But in many urban areas, where trees have been removed and smog has been added, there's no more than 10 percent. We don't breathe as deeply in such an oxygen-poor environment, so each breath provides less oxygen for our blood. Our tap water is also a problem, because it isn't aerated well in the pipes through which it flows, and it must be loaded with chlorine and other additives to make it safe to drink. Finally, proponents of ozone—"prozoners"—say that chemicals used in agriculture and food processing remove many trace elements important for normal health. They have a point in that regard. The net result is a chronic deficiency of oxygen that the prozoners blame for narrowing our arteries, impairing our intelligence, forming stones in our kidneys and gallbladder, and much more.

Ozone is usually administered by a technique called *auto-hemotherapy*. In this process, a quantity of the patient's blood—usually a pint—is removed, mixed with ozone, and returned intravenously. This gaseous ozone mixture can also be injected into muscle, given as an enema for the treatment of diarrhea and local rectal problems, and can even be blown into the vagina to eliminate fungal infections such as candida. (My gynecologist friends shudder at this last application and say it's hazardous, even deadly.) Claims have also been made that ozone is effective against Parkinson's disease, various cancers, and infections, and efficacious in healing wounds.

What's the documentation for all these presumed benefits? Most of the relevant literature on ozone deals with animals and cell cultures, not humans. Back in 1931, Otto Warburg—a doctor and Nobel laureate—first showed that cancer cells differ from their normal counterparts in a fundamental way. Normal cells utilize oxygen and give off carbon dioxide, but cancer cells do the reverse: like plants, they thrive on carbon dioxide and produce oxygen as waste. This observation was confirmed some fifty years later in a study published in *Science*. The growth of human cancer cells from the lungs, breasts, and uterus was shown to be inhibited by nontoxic concentrations of ozone in the test tube; normal cells were unaffected. So, at least theoretically, flooding cancerous tissue with oxygen in the form of ozone should impair its nutrition and arrest its growth. However, most scientists believe the reverse to be true—that extra oxygen actually nourishes cancer cells in the body and speeds their spread.

Although there are scattered reports of cancer patients benefiting from ozone therapy, there are no large, documented studies on this subject. Here is most recent official statement of the American Cancer Society:

> Hyperoxygenation is a method of cancer management based on the erroneous concept that cancer is caused by oxygen-deficiency and can be cured by exposing cancer cells to more oxygen than they can tolerate. Although hyperoxygenating agents have been the subject of legitimate research, there is little or no evidence that they are effective for the treatment of any serious disease, and each has demonstrated potential for harm. Therefore, the American Cancer Society recommends that persons with cancer *not* seek treatment from individuals promoting any form of hyperoxygenation therapy as an "alternative" to proven medical modalities.

Many viruses, especially those with a lipid or fat coating—such as cytomegalus virus, Epstein-Barr virus, and the viruses that cause AIDS, herpes, and hepatitis—are also said to be destroyed when ozone oxidizes the molecules in their coating or shell. Researchers use autohemotherapy to mix ozone with about a pint of the patient's blood. There, its molecules dissolve, releasing their third oxygen atom, which purportedly destroys the virus by attacking its fat shell. The treated blood, now containing antiviral properties, is then returned to the patient. This procedure is performed as often as twice a day, and no less frequently than twice a week. The disease being treated is said to remain under control as long as an "oxygen-positive state" is maintained by means of autohemotherapy and supplemented by exercise, a healthful diet, and proper breathing that moves the oxygen into the lungs.

Doctors in Germany claim to have cured AIDS with autohemotherapy. However, their supporting data, presented to the American scientific community, including Anthony Fauci, the doctor who heads the AIDS program in the United States, were not considered valid or confirmatory. Our scientists raised questions about the accuracy of the diagnosis in the patients who were allegedly cured, as well as the details of their treatment. And so, at least as far as American scientists were concerned, the role of ozone in the treatment of AIDS remained unproved.

Another evaluation of ozone's effectiveness against AIDS was conducted in Canada. The results: "Ozone had no significant effect on hematological, biochemical or clinical toxicity when compared with placebo." In plain language, this means that the ozone, though nontoxic, had no measurable effect on patients with AIDS. The "oxygen community" responded to this negative assessment by claiming that the Canadian researchers had administered the ozone improperly. I was surprised by the reply to this charge and am reproducing in full a public statement by one of the investigators, M. E. Shannon, Canada's deputy surgeon general, which he wrote on January 13, 1995:

> Notwithstanding the negative findings of Dr. Garber's 1991 clinical trial, I firmly believe that ozone therapy has potential

to play a valuable role in the medical management of AIDS. From a regulatory point of view, it is clear that not all forms of ozone therapy will be considered to be sufficiently safe and/or efficacious in this regard; however, there is no doubt in my mind that a protocol will eventually emerge with proven benefit. Looking back at my past experience with autohemotherapy in the treatment of AIDS, there still remains a discrepancy between the phase 1a and 1b trial results (these are preliminary studies done in animals to determine safety and dosage requirements) which may, in part, relate to the lack of sophisticated technology to control for O_3 concentrations (ozone) in both trials. Given the lack of any significant breakthroughs in the treatment of AIDS since that ill-fated trial and the growing testimonial support for its efficacy, the need for further clinical research with ozone is certainly indicated. It is indeed unfortunate that the North American medical community and its funding agencies could not take a more neutral stance on this subject; tragically, professional opinion has been somewhat polarized on this issue. I believe that it is time to take the emotion out of the arguments, both pro and con, and commence a systematic examination of the evidence currently available on the merits of this therapy. Where information gaps exist (particularly in peer-reviewed scientific studies) which might preclude any regulatory decision on the validity of certain claims, properly designed research initiatives should be encouraged with the same kind of public support normally afforded any other scientific endeavor of this import. Although I have my doubts that ozone will ever be shown to have certain curative value in AIDS, I am certain that its well-documented analgesic effects and, hence, its potential impact on patient well-being and quality of life, will someday be recognized. In this regard, I understand that both the FDA and the National Institutes of Health are presently reviewing the scientific merits of ozone as part of their program to investigate a number of "alternative approaches" to AIDS therapy. I have the utmost confidence that in their continued pursuit of an answer to this problem, ozone will receive the scientific attention and support it rightfully deserves.

This statement by a high official of the Canadian government reflects the kind of intellectual honesty and open-mindedness that should guide our decisions, not only with respect to the issue of ozone, but for any kind of therapy that may conceivably help humankind. Given Shannon's strong statement regarding his own research experience with ozone, we should take a more serious look at some of the other claims made for this therapy, the American Cancer Society's current position notwithstanding.

In reviewing the world literature, I came across several references to other uses of ozone that appear to have promise and to warrant further investigation. For example, from Cuba comes a report that intravenous ozone therapy lowers cholesterol levels and stimulates the action of antioxidants in patients with heart disease; from Italy there are claims of improved blood flow in persons with arteriosclerotic disease after ozone therapy; there are studies from Poland attesting to the usefulness of ozone in treating such eye disorders as glaucoma, optic neuritis, and injuries to the cornea; Spanish doctors tell of favorable results in the therapy of chronic leg ulcers. Unfortunately, most of these reports are anecdotal and lack scientific documentation.

Although ozone can be toxic and irritating, it apparently has no significant side effects when properly administered in the recommended doses.

Hydrogen Peroxide

Hydrogen peroxide (H_2O_2) is the stuff many people put on cuts and sores to prevent infections in order to avoid the sting of iodine or alcohol. Formed when ozone (O_3) comes into contact with water, it's yet another way to provide hyperoxygenation. The richest natural source of hydrogen peroxide is atmospheric ozone, so it's abundantly present in rain and snow, especially in unpolluted mountain streams, where the rushing water is constantly aerated and oxygenated. The springwater at Lourdes, in France, which comes from snow melted at high altitudes, where the atmosphere is rich in ozone, is loaded with hydrogen peroxide. (Perhaps that's why, in addition to presumed divine intervention, so many pilgrims feel better when they go to Lourdes.) Hydrogen peroxide is also abundant in raw fruits and vegetables, but most of it is lost when they're cooked. Another natural source of hydrogen peroxide is mother's milk, especially the colostrum present immediately after birth. To stimulate the immune system, the body forms hydrogen peroxide by combining its water content with any oxygen that's available. Scientists theorize that interferon has antiviral and anticancer properties because it increases the formation of hydrogen peroxide.

The available strengths of hydrogen peroxide vary from the 3 percent solution that you can buy over the counter, and even at the grocery store, to the 90 percent grade used to propel rockets. The weaker stuff is perfectly safe to put on scrapes and cuts. However, any concentration greater than 3 percent is potentially dangerous. If you get any of it on your skin, flush it immediately with running water. Should you accidentally ingest concentrated hydrogen peroxide, call your doctor or poison control center right away and start drinking large amounts of water while waiting to go to the emergency room. Ingestion of hydrogen peroxide can be fatal if untreated. Some people drink food-grade 35 percent hydrogen peroxide because they believe it can relieve arthritic pains and other miscellaneous symptoms. I've seen no proof that this is so, and I strongly advise against its use.

Despite criticism from such health icons as the FDA and the American Cancer Society, sales of hydrogen peroxide are increasing in this country by about 15 percent a year. Much of it is bought for uses other than healing, such as for insecticide sprays, for washing laundry and dishes, as an air freshener for the kitchen or bathroom, and as a facial cleanser. But H_2O_2 is also recommended by some "health providers" for the treatment of a host of diseases and symptoms. They believe that hydrogen peroxide, administered in "rejuvenating, detoxifying" baths, foot soaks, mouthwashes, toothpaste, ear drops, nasal sprays, douches, colonics or enemas, by vein—you name it—"selectively kills weak, diseased cells" that the body replaces with new, healthy cells. Such treatment may take several days or weeks. Infections (viral, fungal, and bacterial) are said to respond best, allegedly because hydrogen peroxide stimulates the immune system.

The FDA is not impressed with any of the claims made for hydrogen peroxide in some 5,000 articles, the vast majority of which have appeared in the lay literature and popular magazines, not in scientific journals. It has ruled that hydrogen peroxide in any concentration is *unsafe for human consumption* and may not be sold for "healing" purposes (except for cleansing the skin).

❖ ❖ ❖   What's the bottom line with regard to oxygen therapy?

Hyperbaric oxygen is useful and can even be lifesaving in treating a wide variety of illnesses such as decompression sickness, air embolism, and carbon monoxide poisoning. It may speed the healing of tissues burned or injured by radiation; and it may help in the management of chronic infections, such as those that affect bone (e.g., osteomyelitis). Unfortunately, these chambers are so expensive to buy and maintain that relatively few hospitals have them. Claims for the effectiveness of hyperbaric oxygen against AIDS, cancer, multiple sclerosis, stroke, or Alzheimer's disease are not supported by the evidence. Remember, also, that too much oxygen under pressure, as it is in hyperbaric therapy, can be dangerous, especially for people with chronic lung diseases or ear infections.

Ozone and *hydrogen peroxide* are widely used here and abroad because they are believed to deliver extra oxygen to the tissues. Many claims have been made in the alternative medicine literature for their effectiveness in several disorders, notably cancer, AIDS, and other infections. Although there is no scientifically valid proof, there is enough suggestive evidence to warrant their further study. In the meantime, I personally would not accept ozone therapy, particularly to treat an infection. Results from antibiotics are more predictable. I know of no one with cancer who was cured by ozone (even though it is used at the Gerson clinic in Mexico). However, if I had AIDS, I would be inclined to try ozone because there are no other effective treatments, and some data do suggest that it may make life more tolerable. As far as hydrogen peroxide is concerned, I'd limit it to topical applications for disinfecting purposes. Never take hydrogen peroxide internally for any reason. It can be dangerous and even fatal if ingested, injected, or put into contact with the skin in concentrated form.

❖ 29 ❖

REFLEXOLOGY
Even If You're Ticklish?

Reflexology is a widely accepted form of alternative medicine, with more than 25,000 practitioners worldwide. The technique involves applying pressure to a particular part of the body, most commonly the soles of the feet (but sometimes also the palms, and even the ears). This is believed to send impulses to, and improve the function of, specific organs in the body said to be connected in some way to these pressure sites. Some reflexologists are of the opinion that their technique operates via the same meridians or pathways involved in acupuncture.

Reflexology was used in China as long as 5,000 years ago, and it is depicted in a fresco found in an Egyptian tomb dating back to 2330 B.C. Something very much like reflexology was performed in India long ago, and more recently by some Native Americans.

Reflexology was reintroduced to the West in 1913 by William Fitzgerald, an ear, nose, and throat specialist in

Connecticut. He noted that patients on whom he operated experienced less pain when pressure was applied to their hands, soles, or palms just before surgery. After reproducing this phenomenon in a series of experiments, he concluded that "bioelectrical energy" flows from defined points in the hands and feet to specific zones of the body. Fitzgerald drew complex charts indicating the locations of these points in the feet, and the organs with which they communicate. It is said that applying pressure to such a point produces a positive feedback effect on the corresponding internal organs. For example, the big toe is said to connect directly to the brain; the heel and back of the foot connect to the anus and rectum; the arches lead to the solar plexus.

Reflexology probably would not have gone very far in the modern world had it not been for the efforts of Eunice Ingham, a physiotherapist-masseuse. Despite Fitzgerald's pioneering work, it is Ingham who is considered to be the founder of modern reflexology. Expanding and refining Fitzgerald's observations, she claimed that exerting less pressure, and varying it, not only reduced pain but conferred other health benefits as well.

Practitioners of reflexology assert that they can help 100 conditions or ailments: diarrhea, constipation, and other digestive disorders; stress-related disorders such as migraine and asthma; chronic pain (from arthritis or sciatica); allergic reactions; skin conditions such as acne, psoriasis, and eczema; tension; and neurological symptoms such as those associated with multiple sclerosis. Some reflexologist somewhere is bound to assure you that he or she can fix it.

I've tried reflexology. I love it. It's very relaxing. But I have found that whenever a doctor, or indeed any therapist, "touches" a patient, the patient almost always responds positively. Like a good massage, reflexology leaves you "feeling well." But reflexologists think there's more to what they do than simply a "Dr. Feelgood" effect. They assert that their manipulations are beneficial because of two specific mechanisms. First, they reduce the amount of lactic acid in the tissues of the feet. (Lactic acid is the end product of muscle contraction, a by-product of metabolism which is to the body what exhaust is to the automobile. Too much of it is bad for you.) Second, reflexologists claim that tiny calcium crystals accumulate in the nerve endings of the feet and impede the free flow of "energy" from the local zone to its related organs elsewhere in the body. These crystals are broken up by the therapist's firm compression, which releases toxins and restores "equilibrium."

Most doctors think that this "scientific" explanation is mumbo jumbo. No podiatrist (foot specialist) I know has ever felt such microcrystals, and podiatrists work on feet all day long. Furthermore, I doubt that anyone has ever measured the lactic acid concentration in feet, either before or after reflexology; and I don't know how to define or assess the "energy" whose flow is said to be altered or restored as a result of these manipulations. But most people aren't interested in theory; they want to know whether or not something works. So I have no problem agreeing to or even recommending reflexology for anyone who enjoys it. If you're one of the many thousands who do, be my guest, but don't expect it to melt gallstones or open your coronary arteries.

Reflexology differs from many other forms of alternative medicine in several important ways. Unlike acupuncturists or homeopaths, reflexologists are not doctors and do not usually pretend to be. Most are physiotherapists or masseurs or masseuses with special training in this field. Some spas and health clubs employ full-time reflexologists. However, chances are you'll find—as I did at one health club—that the "reflexologist" and the "masseur" or "masseuse" are one and the same person. My therapist didn't really know anything about specific areas in the feet connecting to target organs in the body—but she did give me a delicious foot massage. At another health club, after the pedicurist had done my toes, she asked me whether I also wanted some reflexology. I consented, and again received a generic nonspecific foot massage.

Some nurses give reflexology instead of sleeping pills to older patients. Midwife reflexologists say that reflexology promotes relaxation during labor, corrects urinary retention, and reduces breast engorgement after delivery. Reflexology is also said to lessen anxiety, especially among the elderly and people who are terminally ill.

The run-of-the-mill reflexologist will treat your symptoms without volunteering an opinion as to what's causing them. This makes it all the more important to establish a proper diagnosis of what ails you before seeking relief from reflexology rather than from a doctor.

A reflexology session usually lasts about forty-five minutes. You sit in a comfortable position with your legs raised while the therapist applies gentle but firm pressure or massage to your feet, using the thumb and fingers in small, creeping, caterpillar-like movements. (Occasionally, reflexologists also use electrical massage, clothespins, rubber balls, elastic bands, and brushes.) An experienced reflexologist claims to be able to tell from the feel of the tissues, and the degree of tenderness, where to focus his or her attention. The usual course of treatment consists of six weekly sessions, depending on the severity and seriousness of your complaints, how long you've had them, the skill of the therapist, and how much time and money you can spend. Several of my patients and friends enjoy reflexology so much and feel so relaxed after receiving it that they have it done every week or two. Being ticklish or having sensitive feet does not preclude this therapy.

Reflexologists tell me that their treatments occasionally produce evidence of a "healing crisis," the nature of which depends on what your problems were in the first place. For example, someone with a respiratory illness may experience a flare-up of cold or flu symptoms; and if the problem is in the gastrointestinal tract, reflexology may worsen diarrhea, flatulence, nausea, or vomiting. Other manifestations of a healing crisis include fever; excess sweating; skin rashes; and a change in the volume, color, or odor of urine. Such crises are said to be due to the release and excretion of accumulated toxins and other waste products, and are alleged to prove that the body is healing itself. A crisis may last for two or three days, but it is followed by a sense of well-being. I could find nothing in the scientific literature to validate these claims.

Reflexology is generally safe, but there are still some precautions you should take. For example, if your feet have been injured in any way, postpone treatment until they've healed. You don't want anyone mashing a cut, bruise, boil, damaged tendon, or recent fracture! Most reflexologists will not treat you if you have a fever (which they interpret as caused by an influx of toxins), or after recent surgery, at least until the incision is healed. I also suggest that you avoid this therapy if you have clots in the veins (deep vein thrombosis or phlebitis), ulcers, or any other vascular problem in your lower legs. If someone has a pacemaker, a reflexologist will usually avoid stimulating the left chest zone; if someone has gallstones or kidney stones, the reflexologist avoids the gallbladder or kidney points in the feet. Also, despite the benefits claimed for pregnant women at or near delivery, my obstetrician colleagues do not think it's a good idea for a pregnant woman to receive reflexology without her doctor's consent, presumably because vigorous pressure to the feet may induce uterine contractions.

I searched the medical literature for objective proof that reflexology does anything more than relax you and found only an occasional reference to it in the mainstream journals. The rest of the material on reflexology appeared in periodicals that did not have the stringent standards for study design and reproducibility that academic, scientific organs apply. However, I did come across one paper, published in December 1993 in *Obstetrics and Gynecology*. It was written jointly by a Ph.D. affiliated with the Division of Behavioral Medicine of the California Graduate Institute in Los Angeles and a reflexologist who belongs to the American Academy of Reflexology. They reviewed the response to reflexology of the ear, hand, and foot in thirty-eight women with premenstrual symptoms. In this randomized, controlled study, the subjects all believed that they were being treated with reflexology. However, half were receiving simple massage not directed at specific points; the others got the "real McCoy," that is, the points massaged on the ears, hands, and feet were selected because of their postulated connection to organs thought to contribute to the symptoms of PMS—the ovaries, the uterus, portions of the nervous system, and various hormone-secreting glands. The two groups reacted differently. Symptoms improved in only 17 percent of those who were simply massaged (although all of them enjoyed the treatment). By contrast, 46 percent of the group treated with reflexology had a definite reduction in the severity of their complaints. This study was conducted in a scientifically acceptable way, but I would like to see it reproduced by other researchers before drawing any conclusions from it.

Reflexology institutes are springing up everywhere. They offer courses to increase proficiency and to certify competence. If you're looking to reflexology to relieve the symptoms of a specific disorder (as opposed to simply getting a good foot massage), find out whether you're being treated by someone who is really trained in the field. In the United States, you can contact the International Institute of Reflexology, P. O. Box 12642, Saint Petersburg, FL 33733; telephone 813-343-4811. This institute is headed by Dwight Byers, a nephew of the late Eunice Ingham and an authority on foot reflexology in his own right.

❖ ❖ ❖ What's the bottom line? I do not usually recommend reflexology to my patients as a medical treatment. If they ask me about it, I tell them exactly what I have written above. And as my mother used to say about so many things, with few exceptions, "Harm, it can't do you." It's okay to try if you are suffering from some chronic, nonthreatening illness—such as irritable bowel, PMS, or migraine—for which there is no other definitive treatment.

❖ 30 ❖

BROWSING IN YOUR
HEALTH FOOD STORE

There's a very well stocked health food store around the corner from my office. I used to go there regularly, but just to buy sesame seed candies, for which I have always had a passion. When I started writing this book, however, and researching all the claims made by practitioners of complementary medicine about the benefits of supplements, herbs, and other products that were exotic to me, I began to scan its shelves with a more discerning eye.

The marketing efficiency of these stores amazes me. Within days after a report appears in the media about a "breakthrough" in alternative therapy for some disease or symptom, their shelves display the cure. If I didn't know better, I'd think these supplies were kept in the basement all along—in anticipation, just waiting for the announcement—and then quickly brought upstairs. Walking through these stores every couple of weeks keeps me posted on what my patients are reading and what they're likely to ask me about. Among the currently popular products are chromium (touted for building better bodies), melatonin (hailed as a cure for jet lag and whatever else ails you), DHEA (which promises to keep you young and healthy), shark cartilage (said to prevent and treat cancer), glucosamine (said to control arthritis), and many others. In this chapter, I will discuss these and other products capturing headlines—and shelf space in health food stores.

Melatonin

Ponce de León may not have found the fountain of youth, but health food stores in this country think they've discovered it in melatonin. Near the cash counter, in the premium selling space, you're likely to see shelf upon shelf of melatonin. I'm told it's now outselling vitamin C, America's number-one vitamin cure-all. Magazine articles, newspaper stories, and best-selling books are all touting melatonin as a miracle drug that can make you live longer and better, make you sexier, let you sleep more soundly, and protect you against almost every disorder from jet lag to cancer. I learned long ago that anything that sounds too good to be true probably isn't. Here, stripped of the hype, are the *facts* about melatonin.

Melatonin is not an herb or a natural food. It's a hormone produced by the pineal gland, an organ the size of a pea located in the middle of the brain behind the eyes. Melatonin structurally resembles the amino acid tryptophan, a sleep aid that was once available—as melatonin is now—without a doctor's prescription. (Tryptophan was pulled from the market after thirty-eight people died from some batches that had been contaminated in the manufacturing process.) Like tryptophan, melatonin promotes sleep. The body, in its wisdom, makes most of its melatonin during the night, when we want to sleep, though as we get older the brain produces less and less melatonin (this is why older folks don't sleep as much or as soundly as babies). But helping you get to sleep is only the most apparent and obvious effect of melatonin; it also interacts in very complicated ways with virtually every other hormone in the body, and with a network of chemicals (serotonin is one of the more important ones) that influence everything from behavior to the immune system. None of the body's chemical constituents operates in a vacuum, so if you introduce extra amounts of one chemical, nature compensates by making less of some (or all) of the others. Therefore, taking melatonin as regularly as you would a vitamin (which many of its proponents suggest) may disturb the inner equilibrium of the body, with unpredictable long-term effects. Advertising and selling melatonin in supermarkets and health food stores, without restrictions, warnings, and responsible instructions for dosages, makes about as much sense as offering estrogen, testosterone, insulin, or any other potent hormone to children in a candy store. But such are the vagaries of the drug regulatory process in this country.

Although there have been many studies of the immediate biological effects of melatonin in humans, most have been carried out in animals and their results have been extrapolated to humans. For example, mice who had been rendered susceptible to cancer were given melatonin every night after the age of one month (the amount was the equivalent of 3 milligrams in a human). Sixty-seven percent of the untreated animals in the study went on to develop cancer, but only 23 percent of those who had been given melatonin did so. In another animal study, very small doses of melatonin protected experimental animals from the toxic effects of radiation. In other research, melatonin was found to increase the production of antibodies in laboratory animals.

Melatonin is a powerful antioxidant in mice, neutralizing oxygen-free radicals that are the end result of many energy processes in the body; these radicals are thought to promote aging, accelerate arteriosclerosis, and reduce immunity. In one experiment, when the pineal glands (where melatonin is made) of old mice and young mice were switched, the "seniors" appeared rejuvenated in every way, while the "youngsters" aged very quickly. Unfortunately, there's no way to duplicate this experiment with human subjects. (If you know of any volunteers, please get in touch with me immediately.)

Does melatonin prevent or fight cancer in humans? Some experimental work done with human subjects suggests that powerful antioxidants like melatonin can prevent the damage to DNA caused by oxygen-free radicals—damage that can leave us more vulnerable to cancer. Also, there is a chemical in the body called interleukin-2 that slows down the production of tumor growth factor. When animals with cancer are given melatonin and interleukin-2, the malignant process appears to slow down. In 1995, researchers reported that in human subjects, melatonin also reduces the properties of estrogen that stimulate the growth of tumors; and that it blocks the action of prolactin, a tumor-promoting hormone made in the brain.

These are just some of the theoretical and experimental data concerning melatonin. There is much more, enough to fill a few best-selling books. Here, for practical purposes, is what it boils down to at present.

• *Jet lag.* I travel a great deal, often across time zones, and I have found melatonin extremely effective in preventing jet lag. I take 2 or 3 milligrams just after I board the plane. Then I have another 2 milligrams at bedtime for the next two or three days until I've adjusted to the new time zone.

- *Sleep.* Melatonin is probably safe for occasional use, no more often than once or twice a week, to help you get a good night's sleep. The usual dosage is 2 or 3 milligrams (the strength you're most likely to find at a health food store or pharmacy), but this amount is strictly empirical: there is no "officially" recommended dose. Some observers report success with as little as half a milligram at bedtime. Many of my patients who have used melatonin for this purpose tell me that it works and does not appear to be habituating. But it frequently induces vivid dreams and nightmares, often frightening enough to discourage its use. I have tried it myself, and I can tell you that the nightmares are real—so real, in fact, that unless I'm traveling, I'd rather spend a sleepless night than endure them.

- *Tumors.* Given the experimental evidence for the possible anticancer effects of melatonin, I have no hesitation about recommending it in combination with interleukin-2 to patients with advanced tumors of the reproductive organs such as the ovaries, testes, breasts, and adrenal glands— under a doctor's supervision, of course. However, I do not recommend melatonin for preventing cancer, given how little we know of its long-term effects in healthy people.

- *Aging.* I have seen no convincing evidence of any properties in melatonin that would prevent aging.

- *Contraindications.* Most scientists recommend that you not take melatonin if you have an *autoimmune disorder* such as lupus or rheumatoid arthritis (ask your doctor whether the condition for which he or she is treating you falls into that category), *lymphoma, leukemia,* or *severe allergies,* or if you are *pregnant* or *nursing*—again, because many of its subtle and long-term actions remain unknown. And don't give it your kids either. They have enough of their own, and you don't want to meddle with their *milieu intérieur.*

• *Caveat.* Whenever you buy melatonin, look at the label to see how and where it's made. Most brands in the United States are synthetic, but some imported products may be derived from animal pineal glands. What with the concern about mad cow disease, you're better off avoiding these "natural" products.

❖ ❖ ❖ The bottom line? With the exception of some documented late-stage malignancies, I recommend melatonin only for intermittent, temporary use. That's because its long-term safety has not been established, and many of its alleged benefits have thus far been shown to occur only in animals.

DHEA

DHEA—dehydroepiandrosterone—is another of those all-encompassing "miracle" hormones currently drawing considerable attention from scientists and the lay public. I predict that you'll be hearing lots more about this one in the future. DHEA, made by the adrenal glands, which sit on top of the kidneys, is often referred to as the "mother hormone" because it is the precursor to steroid hormones, adrenaline, and several other hormones, including estrogen and testosterone. Although promoted mainly for its antiaging effect, it is said to have many other benefits too.

I have reviewed the data in more than 2,000 references to DHEA in the medical literature. Much of the research has been done by credible scientists such as Etienne Emile Beaulieu, the French Nobel laureate who discovered melatonin, and I found a mixture of excitement and uncertainty.

There were several reports attesting to the *potential* of DHEA to improve sexual function; build muscle mass (especially in the elderly); reduce the incidence of such diseases as arteriosclerosis, cancer, autoimmune disorders, osteoporosis, Alzheimer's, chronic fatigue syndrome, depression, and herpes; and reduce the ravages of stress. It appears that many people affected with various conditions have lower levels of DHEA than healthy people of the same age and sex. In one study, for example, of 5,000 women followed over a five-year period, all those with DHEA levels at least 10 percent lower than normal for their age developed and died of breast cancer. Conversely, every woman whose DHEA was higher than average remained free of cancer. The same association was found for heart disease. In a study at the University of California at San Diego, the DHEA levels of 242 men between the ages of fifty and seventy-nine were monitored for twelve years. Men with low DHEA levels had twice the incidence of heart disease and death as men whose DHEA was high. Similar results were obtained for most of the other disorders listed above. Optimists and pessimists will react differently to these data. The optimists will conclude that supplemental DHEA prevents, slows, or reverses breast cancer and heart disease. Pessimists will argue that low DHEA levels could very well be an *effect* of disease rather than a cause. They can point out, for example, that bacterial pneumonia is associated with a high white-blood-cell count, but that is not the cause of the lung infection!

In the laboratory, rats rendered cancer-prone and then treated with DHEA developed cancer much less frequently than cancer-prone rats left untreated. Rabbits that were force-fed diets high in saturated fat uniformly developed arteriosclerotic plaques in their blood vessels—the fatty buildup associated with heart disease. But rabbits pretreated with DHEA had plaques only half the size of those in the untreated control group.

◆ ◆ ◆

One day in 1996, one of my patients asked me to write him a prescription for DHEA as soon as possible—he had just read a piece about it in *Vanity Fair*. The article that so excited my patient presented all the positive findings mentioned above. But the author did not mention other, adverse findings. For example, in the heart study I described above, *women* with high DHEA levels turned out to be at *greater* risk of heart disease! What's more, when the male subjects were followed for longer than twelve years, the protective effect of DHEA did not persist. The doctor who conducted these studies—Elizabeth Barret-Connor, a distinguished researcher—recently wrote in *The Sciences* that she was surprised that "physicians out there are giving this drug to thousands of people" without really knowing enough about it. Because of its relationship to the male hormone testosterone, DHEA can cause acne and facial hair in women; and it can cause insulin resistance in both sexes. In another experiment with rats, among sixteen that had been given DHEA, fourteen developed cancer of the liver. This would probably be enough to stop DHEA testing in humans, if DHEA were a drug rather than a supplement.

The *Vanity Fair* piece is typical of the hype that accompanies discussions of antiaging and other "miracle" drugs. Some of these agents, including DHEA, may very well turn out to be everything that their proponents claim. I hope so. But there's lots more research to be done first. Proper dosages must be determined in women and men, and long-term studies must be carried out. Unfortunately, because DHEA is a natural substance and cannot be patented, the drug industry is not motivated to invest the large sums of money required for such research. Instead, the industry is looking for synthetic derivatives.

* ◆ *

One of my physician friends is very keen on DHEA. After participating in some of its early clinical studies, he was so impressed with the results that he now prescribes it for virtually every patient over age fifty. The last time we had a drink together, a few months ago, he persuaded me to try some. "I promise you'll feel terrific—half your age. You'll thank me, and so will your wife." (Of course, I had no idea what my wife had to do with it. She could very well take her own, couldn't she?) "But first I'll need to get some blood tests on you. Have your technician draw seven tubes, and send them over. We'll do the rest." He went on to extol the antiaging effects of DHEA. He explained to me that DHEA is highest early in life; by age forty it's only half of what it was at age twenty-one; by age sixty-five, only one-tenth; and by age eighty, only one-twentieth. And that, he was certain, is why we age. He reminded me that although life expectancy in this country has risen to approximately eighty years (from about fifty years at the turn of the century), we still begin to "get older" as we enter middle age. By the time we reach fifty, most of us are a little flabby, we don't hear or see as well, our sex drive and performance abate, our metabolism slows, our skin becomes wrinkled, and we start to get paunchy. According to my friend, DHEA turns the clock back for all these physical and physiological midlife changes.

Although I was feeling perfectly well, I wanted to stay that way. So I signed on for DHEA. My friend gave me my first bottle, which contained a hundred 50-milligram tablets. He told me to take one tablet daily (the currently recommended dose) and assured me that I'd have no side effects. (He was apparently selling DHEA to his patients because at the time it was hard to find. The regulatory agencies were treating it as a restricted drug whose safety and effectiveness had not been proven; you couldn't buy it at health food stores after the FDA banned its sale in 1985, and most pharmacies weren't stocking it.)

After taking DHEA for about a month, I couldn't honestly say I felt any different. (My wife noticed no change, either.) I reported this to my doctor friend, and he encouraged me to stay with it. At the end of the second month, I was having trouble sleeping; but I had a lot on my mind at the time, so I wasn't sure this was due to the DHEA. At just about that time, I learned the results of my blood tests—which, incidentally cost over $400. (Medicare—I'm over sixty-five, but I certainly don't look it—wouldn't pay for them. "Not medically necessary" was their reasoning.) My friend was amazed at my test results. My DHEA level, before the supplements, was that of a thirty-year-old! Maybe that's why I hadn't responded more dramatically to this hormone. In any event, given the excellent amount of DHEA in my bloodstream, I stopped taking it. Now I am sleeping well again (no one else I know on DHEA has complained of insomnia), and I feel younger than ever. So that's one man's experience with this hormone. I suppose that the only fair conclusion is that if you're going to try DHEA, get your blood levels checked first—and negotiate the lab fee in advance!

I am cautious about recommending or prescribing DHEA in my practice. I advise men with prostate cancer not to take it, since the body converts it to testosterone, which can make the tumor more aggressive. Because DHEA is a precursor of estrogen, I believe that women who have a strong family history of cancer of the breast or ovaries, or who have already developed such a malignancy, should also avoid it. Someone under age forty who takes it may cause his or her own body to stop making it naturally, with unknown consequences. Whenever you're tempted to jump onto the bandwagon of any untested medication, always remember the examples of

radiation and antibiotics. These have been extremely important advances in the history of medicine—lifesaving when
used properly. But they are potentially life-threatening
when misapplied or given in the wrong doses; it took years
of study to determine when they should be used and in what
amounts. That information is not yet on hand for DHEA.

So what's the bottom line on taking DHEA now? If you
decide to "jump the gun" and use it (against my advice),
make sure to have your DHEA level checked before you do so
to see whether it's truly low. And don't take DHEA under
any circumstances if you're under forty or if you have have
prostate, breast, or ovarian cancer. Finally, although DHEA
may turn out to be a "miracle" drug against aging and a variety of serious diseases, remember that it is a powerful hormone whose safety and effectiveness have not been proven.

Coenzyme Q10

You'll find Coenzyme Q10—ubiquinone, also known as
CoQ10—in every health food store, alone or in combination
with a host of other vitamins. CoQ10 is a vitamin-like substance, a naturally occurring antioxidant made mostly by
the liver but also derived from food (especially meat). In
addition to scavenging oxygen-free radicals in the human
cell, as all antioxidants do, it produces ATP, the energy molecule that powers many cellular reactions in our body.
CoQ10 is a very big item in Japan, where I understand some
6 million people take it regularly, as do a substantial number in this country. To keep up with the worldwide demand,
some eighty pharmaceutical companies manufacture it
alone or in combination with vitamins, minerals, and other
chemicals. Doses vary, because the "correct" dose has never
been established.

CoQ10 is said to have an especially salutary effect on the
heart, and it is often prescribed by alternative physicians for

the treatment of congestive heart failure because it is believed to strengthen heart muscle. Some surgeons give it for that reason to patients who are about to undergo heart surgery. The toxicity to the heart of Adriamycin, a potent anticancer drug, is said to be reduced when CoQ10 is administered along with it. However, despite reports in the scientific literature attesting to these effects (most of which appear in the European literature), the American Heart Association continues to maintain that CoQ10 is still experimental. Proponents of CoQ10 also claim that it stimulates immune function, heals gastric ulcers, promotes weight loss if you're obese, alleviates diabetes and muscular dystrophy, strengthens the gums, and enhances physical performance, such as athletic activity.

One problem with obtaining substantial research data on CoQ10 is similar to what I described for DHEA; both are natural substances that cannot be patented, and thus there is no financial incentive for drug companies to engage in long and costly research. Such research might benefit not only humanity but also competitors who have made no investment.

I did come across one interesting and possibly important study on CoQ10. In 1993, a clinic in Denmark reported that in two women with widely metastasized breast cancer, all traces of malignancy disappeared after they took 390 milligrams of CoQ10 daily for several months. The following year, three more such "cures" were observed. Now, I have no idea what else these patients were being given, or how many others were treated similarly in whom no benefit was noted. A report of only five cases, without double-blind controls (see chapter 2) and without the other requisites of a valid study, is not taken seriously in the scientific community. But for a practicing doctor like me, whose main interest is the one-on-one relationship with my patients, it is very exciting. You can be sure that from now on I will add CoQ10 to the regimen of all my patients who have breast cancer, since I am not aware of any toxicity from this substance.

❖ ❖ ❖   What's the bottom line? CoQ10 is an important natural substance being taken by millions of people for a variety of diseases, but mainly for strengthening the heart. At this time, I have no qualms about letting anyone take it, for whatever reason, particularly since there is no downside of which I am aware. Reports of "cures" of advanced breast cancer should be followed up by the "cancer establishment" even without commercial funding. If you decide to take CoQ10, do so along with your other standard therapy, not as a replacement—and always under your doctor's supervision.

Glucosamine

Some of my patients have been asking me about glucosamine, advertised as a treatment for arthritis, particularly the wear-and-tear form called osteoarthritis that usually involves the back and weight-bearing joints such as the hips and knees.

Conventional therapy for osteoarthritis is not very satisfactory. It consists essentially of a combination of rest and exercise, physiotherapy, massage, heat or cold, weight loss if necessary, and, in the final analysis, painkillers. The latter range from simple aspirin to the more potent nonsteroidal anti-inflammatory drugs such as ibuprofen and related chemicals. The problem with all of the more powerful medications is that their long-term use can cause side effects— gastrointestinal bleeding in the elderly, liver damage, and kidney disorders.

Glucosamine is a water-soluble amino sugar derived from glucose. It is a building block of mucopolysaccharides, compounds present—in a healthy person—in the membranes, ligaments, tendons, and cartilage that make up the joints, as well as the fluid that bathes and lubricates them ("synovial" fluid). When there is a deficiency in glucosamine, this synovial fluid becomes thin and watery and can no longer effectively lubricate and cushion all the moving parts in the joint. According to some researchers, supplemental glucosamine thickens the fluid that bathes the joints, repairs damaged cartilage, relieves pain, and retards the process of osteoarthritis.

I know of no "conventional" doctor who prescribes glucosamine to arthritic patients, despite several studies attesting to its efficacy. Two reports of which I am aware, both from the European literature, are impressive. One study—a double-blind design—involved forty patients with osteoarthritis of the knee. Twenty were given 500 milligrams of glucosamine three times a day; the other twenty received daily doses of 1.2 grams of ibuprofen, a nonsteroidal anti-inflammatory drug. (The latter is the equivalent of six tablets of the over-the-counter drug Advil.) In the first two weeks, the patients on ibuprofen had less pain; but by the end of the eighth week, those in the glucosamine-treated group had greater joint mobility and less pain. Glucosamine yielded similar favorable results in a study of thirty Italian patients with chronic osteoarthritis. These and other researchers recommend taking glucosamine early in the course of arthritis, to prevent or delay its progress. Other papers, reporting similar results, have been published in such mainstream medical journals as *The Lancet* and the *Journal of Bone and Joint Surgery*. I am not aware of any negative reports on glucosamine and have not seen any reports of toxicity.

❖ ❖ ❖   The bottom line on glucosamine? Aspirin and related anti-inflammatory drugs should be used when necessary for relief of pain in osteoarthritis, but it is reasonable to add glucosamine to the therapy. It does not appear to have a downside, except that people with diabetes should avoid it because it is an amino sugar and thus can affect blood sugar.

Chromium

Chromium is another product prominently displayed in health food stores. Some brochures promise that it will increase your muscle mass, lower your cholesterol, reduce your weight, eliminate some of your body fat, and, if you're diabetic, keep your blood sugar on an even keel. One manufacturer of chromium paid a $1.45 million fine for making these claims, not necessarily because they were false or exaggerated but because the company had no right to make them without subjecting its product to the formal testing demanded by the FDA. The most widely advertised of the various chromium preparations is chromium picolinate, and its manufacturers are very circumspect about their claims. Still, there are many people who tout many potential benefits of chromium. Are they right?

A few years ago, a friend of mine, Jeffrey Fisher—a doctor who is a pathologist by training and a very good nutritionist as well—wrote a book called *The Chromium Program* (Harper & Row, 1990). In this book, he reviewed the world literature on chromium and argued that this mineral had potential for good, especially in people with diabetes. He showed me his manuscript and, after I'd finished reading it, invited me to comment on it for publicity purposes. I agreed to do so because I believed at the time that this substance had promise, and I was eager to see further studies done with it. Several years have passed, and this is a good time to evaluate the research that has been done in the interval. It goes without saying that neither Fisher nor I have a vested interest—professional or commercial—in chromium.

◆ ◆ ◆

Chromium is a trace mineral that is needed for many body functions, but in only tiny amounts. Its most important role, from which many of its effects stem, is increasing the effectiveness of insulin, which helps regulate blood sugar levels and metabolizes fat. Insulin is also believed to increase muscle mass as it decreases fat deposits. Chromium therefore is often called the "insulin cofactor." Under normal circumstances, your tissues store only enough fat in reserve to tide you over periods of nutritional deprivation and to insulate various body organs. Some people, including diabetics, develop insulin resistance, a condition in which the cells do not permit insulin to enter and metabolize fat. This leads to excess storage of fat—and obesity. Chromium reduces insulin resistance, increases fat metabolism, and prevents fat from accumulating. In other words, thanks to chromium we are less likely to gain (fat) weight.

We don't need much chromium in our diet to do the job. Although there's no official RDA, most researchers think that 100 micrograms a day is probably optimal. (By contrast, the estimated average daily intake is 33 micrograms for men and 25 micrograms for women.) However, there are those who think that adolescents and very active people should have as much as 200 micrograms daily. The richest nutritional sources of chromium are brewer's yeast, calves' liver, beef, chicken, shellfish, apples, vegetables (especially potato skins), whole-wheat products, prunes, American cheese, and a variety of spices. In fact, chromium is so abundant that I find it hard to explain the statistics showing that most Americans get so little of it.

Of course, people on intravenous therapy, who aren't taking any food by mouth—and people on crash diets—do lack chromium. Also, the chromium in food is partially lost in cooking and in commercial processing, when germ and bran are removed from whole grains, and when raw sugar is refined. People can also become deficient in chromium if their produce and grains come from chromium-depleted soil, if they drink too much alcohol, and—believe it or not—if they exercise too vigorously. So chromium deficiency is possible; but true chromium deficiency is not very common, and only in the case of a true deficiency would you require or benefit from supplementation.

At the time when Fisher wrote *The Chromium Program,* the data suggested that supplemental chromium would enhance the utilization of insulin by the body. Since then, this has sometimes, *but not always,* been shown to be the case. Despite its effect on the utilization of fat, there have been mixed reports as to whether supplemental chromium speeds fat loss. Some studies conclude that it does, others that it does not. Although there have been papers documenting improved strength and performance among athletes taking chromium, the most recent research I have read reported no difference in burning fat, building muscles, or losing weight between those who took chromium supplements and those who didn't. However, in type 2 diabetes—the adult form in which the insulin produced by the pancreas isn't properly utilized—chromium, either as a supplement or in the diet, does help control blood sugar. I usually prescribe a daily 200-microgram supplement for such diabetics.

There is credible evidence that chromium can lower cholesterol levels somewhat, and it does increase HDL—"good" cholesterol. However, if you have a real cholesterol problem, you'll probably need more specific and more effective therapy to normalize your blood fats.

The most widely advertised chromium supplement is the picolinate form, which is absorbed much more efficiently than other preparations. However, if you are one of those people who believe that if one capsule is good, five must be better, be aware that too much chromium can damage the liver, kidneys, and nerves and disturb heart rhythm. There have been recent reports that excess chromium picolinate in animals can cause cancer, but the doses used were so very high that I don't believe we can extrapolate this effect to humans.

❖ ❖ ❖ So what's the bottom line on chromium? On the basis of my own experience and my review of the latest available literature, I believe that chromium supplements can be of help to people with type 2 diabetes. I see no harm in athletes (or even the elderly) taking chromium supplements (but no more than 200 micrograms per day) to increase muscle mass, since some (though not all) studies show that it may have this effect. Overall, however, supplemental chromium is not necessary for the great majority of people: the body's requirement is very low and is easily satisfied by the average diet.

Shark Cartilage

Shark cartilage is one item you can't miss as you peruse the shelves of your health food store. People are buying it for whatever ails them, but mostly because it's been said to control cancer and to a lesser extent arthritis. There has been enough suggestive evidence for the National Institutes of Health to launch a formal study of the anticancer properties of shark cartilage. (I suspect that public opinion—molded to some extent by programs such as *60 Minutes* on CBS—provided some extra incentive for this funding.)

The concept of using shark cartilage to treat cancer and arthritis stems from the shark's hardiness. The shark, which predates even the dinosaur, has survived the rigors of evolution. It has no bones, only cartilage, the constituents of which are thought to stimulate the immune system. Also, cancers need a constantly increasing blood supply to nourish their wildly growing cells. Shark cartilage blocks the formation of new blood vessels, a process called angiogenesis. So by cutting off a cancer's blood supply, shark cartilage can, at least theoretically, slow or arrest its growth.

The relationship between angiogenesis and the ability of a cancer to spread is more than theoretical. There are some preliminary data documenting an anticancer effect and prolonged survival in people with cancer of the prostate, breast, liver, bone, ovaries, and uterus. Shark cartilage also appeared to help several patients who had developed disorders such as arthritis and psoriasis after conventional chemotherapy and radiation had damaged their immune system. However, because shark cartilage impairs blood supply, you should *not* take it in circumstances when the body needs more blood, for example, if you have a disease of the heart or blood vessels, are pregnant, or are recovering after surgery.

If you're thinking about taking shark cartilage, here are some additional facts you should know. On the positive side, I am not aware of any toxicity from its use. However, many researchers doubt its effectiveness when taken by mouth because the cartilage is digested by the stomach acid before it is absorbed. Under these circumstances, it would seem more reasonable to take it via an enema. Most people would not find that convenient or desirable—and at any rate, other researchers have concluded that the oral route does work.

Be sure you know the source of your shark cartilage, regardless of how you take it. Large supplies of dried sharks' fins and other products have been confiscated at the point of entry into the United States and in warehouses because of contamination with filth and animal excrement. And even if you're convinced that shark cartilage is all it's cracked up to be, do *not* abandon any of your other treatments against cancer or arthritis. As enticing as they are, none of the claims for shark cartilage has been confirmed.

❖ ❖ ❖   What's the bottom line concerning shark cartilage? It has interesting possibilities, but all the facts are not
yet in. Anything more than cautious optimism is premature.
The products used appear so far to be safe; the only danger
lies in abandoning conventional therapy for a pig in a poke.

Boron

I also get asked a lot of questions about boron. I found bottles of boron at the very top of the first shelf in my neigh-
borhood health food store. There is a strategy to these
displays. Goods that are currently "hot" are at eye level and
within easy reach. So the fact that you can't easily pluck
boron off the shelf suggests to me that it's not a big seller.
But the store does stock it, so someone must be buying it. If
that someone is you, here's what you should know about
boron.

Boron is a trace mineral present in leafy vegetables,
apples, raisins, grapes, nuts, and grains. The average American eats between 1 and 2 milligrams of boron per day. Boron
was never a major player in the nutritional game until one
day—some years ago—a report appeared in which women
forty-eight to eighty-two years of age who took 3 milligrams
of supplemental boron a day excreted *smaller* amounts of
calcium, magnesium, and phosphorus in their urine. Since
most of the calcium in urine comes from bone, extra
amounts of boron should presumably result in stronger
bones, and this possibility is especially important for
menopausal women. Boron deficiency is associated not only
with excessive loss of calcium in the urine, but also with
decreased production of estrogen and testosterone and a
higher incidence of arthritis.

What did the health food industry conclude from this? Not
that we should all try to get at least 2 milligrams of boron
a day from fruits and vegetables, but that we need a daily

3-milligram *tablet*. That's how boron got to my (and your) health food store. (I suspect that it may be moved to a more accessible shelf soon, because I found a flyer on the cash counter that read, "Buy three- or six-milligram boron tablets. TAKE ONE A DAY. You should notice a SMALL MIRACLE IN MENTAL ALERTNESS in a few weeks." The difference between a "small" miracle and a "big" miracle was not clarified.)

What's wrong with taking a 3-milligram boron supplement to strengthen your bones if you're menopausal, or to prevent arthritis, or—as athletes say it will—to build muscles and increase stamina? The problem is that menopausal problems, arthritis, or insufficient musculature or stamina do not result from lack of one specific, isolated nutrient. Such conditions are complex and have many causes. I am not aware of any studies demonstrating that menopausal women who have osteoporosis are selectively deficient in boron, so taking boron capsules for that reason makes no sense. There have been some reports that 9 to 10 milligrams of boron a day may help in the treatment of rheumatoid arthritis, especially in children, but doses that high should be taken only under close medical supervision. I haven't found any studies confirming a role for boron in building muscles. Moreover, in addition to its cost and its inconvenience, no one knows how boron interacts with other supplements—of which there are literally thousands.

Too much boron can be toxic; in fact, boron supplements are banned in Australia, despite the fact that boron levels there are low. Although three milligrams a day appears to be safe, I wouldn't exceed that amount, because there have not been any long-term studies documenting the safety of higher doses.

❖ ❖ ❖   The bottom line on boron? Don't bother getting a stepladder to reach the boron on the top shelf. Just eat at least five servings of fruit and vegetables, and have a bowl of cereal in the morning. If you have osteoporosis, review with your doctor the many new ways to maintain and restore the calcium content of your bone.

Royal Jelly

Royal jelly is big business. A creation of the health food industry, it's sold in health food shops everywhere. Although you may run across an endorsement here and there from some "authority," I know of no physician (conventional or complementary) who seriously recommends royal jelly for any ailment. Yes, as do so many other natural products, it contains proteins, minerals, sugar, and fat. But if you happen to be deficient in any of them for whatever reason, you can obtain them much less expensively in other supplements.

Mystique, not science, is what sells royal jelly. It all started when someone took a close look at the feeding and breeding habits of the bee. Royal jelly is the thick, milky-white substance that young (six- to twelve-week-old) worker bees (also called "nurse bees") secrete from glands in their throat. Their purpose in life is to feed this material to young queen bees, and when they do—wow! The queens grow to twice the size of any other bee, they lay 2,000 eggs a day (no small feat), and they live forty times longer than do worker bees. For some people, the natural conclusion is that what's good for bees must be good for humans too. And so they started selling the stuff to gullible females in 100-milligram capsules for about a quarter apiece, and adding it to creams and ointments. The promise? It will reduce the symptoms of PMS, raise the energy level, and (the usual claim) "stimulate the immune system." (Frankly, I would have thought the royal jelly enthusiasts would have been better advised to direct their attention to chickens, whose breeders would love their hens to be twice the size and lay 2,000 eggs a day. The women with whom I have discussed these two potential benefits of royal jelly have no interest in them.) In any event, I could find no evidence whatsoever, aside from its admittedly high concentration of vitamin B, that royal jelly is useful in the prevention or treatment of any human symptoms or disease.

Not only is there no apparent benefit from consuming royal jelly, in some people it can provoke a life-threatening allergic reaction. Several studies have appeared documenting this hazard, and it's not clear what allergen in the royal jelly is responsible for this dangerous response. In most cases of allergy, you must first be sensitized to some substance. Then, when you are exposed to it a second time, that's when the fireworks begin. But several allergic reactions to royal jelly have occurred on the first exposure. So if you happen to be an allergic individual, especially to pollen, don't get involved with royal jelly.

❖ ❖ ❖   The bottom line? Leave royal jelly to the queen bees.

Bee Pollen

Bee pollen is a combination of pollens and nectar—collected by worker bees as they buzz among the flowers—mixed together with the bees' saliva. They carry it on their legs into the hives, where they pack and store it in wax cells. Enter the "nurse bees" described above. They synthesize the bee pollen into a high-protein food (royal jelly), which is then fed to developing larvae and queen bees. Beekeepers interested in marketing bee pollen have devised several ingenious ways of getting it. Some build a trap at the entrance to the hive and remove the pollen from the legs of the honeybees before they enter; some swipe the pollen from the hives after it's been delivered.

And that's how it would have remained had it not been for testimonials by some athletes that bee pollen tablets greatly enhanced their performance—although scientific evaluation of these claims has failed to substantiate them. Another boost for bee pollen was the enthusiasm of Senator Tom Harkin of Iowa. Intelligent and articulate, Senator Harkin is convinced that bee pollen capsules cured his hay fever. There are some who say that this belief was the driving force and main reason behind the establishment by the National Institutes of Health of the Office of Alternative Medicine. Its charge? To fund investigation of all promising "alternative methods, including bee pollen." Despite the dearth of any data showing that bee pollen has any therapeutic value, it remains a popular item in health food stores. Although it is rich in carbohydrates and trace nutrients, few serious practitioners prescribe it for any ailment. Again, as with royal jelly, there are less expensive ways to buy its ingredients. (Bee pollen tablets will run you anywhere from a nickel to fifty cents apiece, depending on whether the pollen is domestic or imported.)

You will hear and read that bee pollen is useful in infections (the truth is that bacteria, yeast, and fungi actually *thrive* on bee pollen, and are not destroyed by it); that it slows the aging process (in support of this claim its proponents point to the long-lived inhabitants of the Caucasus in Georgia—a legend that was widespread for years until someone studied the eating habits of these people and found no evidence that they consumed bee pollen); that bee pollen can relieve the symptoms of allergy (anecdotal, never proved, and, as I indicated above, the reverse can be true); that it is the richest source of protein (its major constituent

happens to be carbohydrate, not protein). For all these reasons, the FDA has ruled that although bee pollen may be
sold as a food supplement, its manufacturers are constrained against claiming that it cures or alleviates any illness, or that it has any therapeutic effect. This decision has
been upheld in the courts and remains in force today.

Like royal jelly, bee pollen can trigger serious allergic
reactions, especially in people who are allergic to pollen,
and the preparations vary in pollen content. So even if you
tolerate one preparation, another may do you in.

❖ ❖ ❖ The bottom line? With all due respect to Senator
Harkin, I advise you to spend your money on honey. Bee
pollen won't do anything for you, and if you're allergic, it
can hurt.

Lecithin

Lecithin is a phospholipid (one of several nutrients consisting of fats, oils, and waxes) called phosphatidyl choline. Its
potential use in treating patients with Alzheimer's disease
is based on the observation that it is needed for normal
brain development in infants and children. Its richest
dietary sources are high-fat, high-cholesterol foods such as
eggs, red meat, and organ meats like liver—not exactly what
you would wish to consume in large amounts. Fortunately,
the lecithin you buy is made from defatted soybean oil. The
problem with most commercial preparations, though, is that
the oil tends to become rancid unless it's packaged in an
oxygen-free container and refrigerated as soon as it is
opened.

Lecithin is a big item in every health food store I've ever
browsed through. Many of my patients take it regularly
because they have read somewhere, or have been told, that

it's great for memory and that it lowers cholesterol. One of them, a man of seventy-five, has been using lecithin (and following a low-fat diet) for three years. Before this regimen, his cholesterol level was about 250 milligrams; it's now 210. Was it the diet or the lecithin—or both? Another patient, a woman of sixty-four, had a cholesterol level of 285 milligrams. She, too, went on a low-fat, low-cholesterol diet and started taking lecithin. Within three months, her cholesterol *rose* to 290 milligrams. These two contrasting cases, in my own practice, prompted me to review the literature to learn what other doctors have found. Although there is a difference of opinion, the nays outnumber the yeas. What's more, the credentials of the naysayers are more impressive than those of the yea-sayers.

For example, Adele Davis, a nutritionist with only so-so scientific credentials, describes experimental studies in which rabbits fed huge amounts of fats uniformly developed atherosclerosis (obstructing arterial plaques) except when they were given lecithin. The problem is that rabbits are not people, and that no one, not even the most gluttonous among us, eats that kind of diet. Fair enough, so Ms. Davis reports that "supplements of lecithin have also caused angina pains to disappear and have been especially helpful to elderly patients who have suffered stroke, or have cerebral atherosclerosis." This observation was made by a physician, Lester Morrison, and published in the journal *Geriatrics* in 1958. To the best of my knowledge, it has never been confirmed. (I knew Lester Morrison. He was an innovative thinker, and postulated way back then that shark cartilage was useful in the treatment of cancer and heart disease.) I find it interesting that most of the sales pitches for lecithin—appearing mostly in publications dealing with alternative medicine and in materials put out by health food distributors—quote this study, which was done almost forty years ago. There has been little, if any, convincing documentation in the scientific literature since that time. Indeed, I must conclude, as does Dr. Joe D. Goldstritch in his book *The Cardiologist's Painless Prescription for a Healthy Heart and Longer Life* (9-Heart-9 Publishing, Dallas, Texas, 1994), "I was hoping to find documentation of lecithin's benefits so I would have still another effective natural therapy to recommend to you. Unfortunately, there is no convincing evidence that lecithin does anything useful. Save your money." (Unfortunately, Goldstritch concludes this paragraph with the following: "It will be much better spent on antioxidants such as vitamins E and C and beta carotene." I'm not sure I endorse that finale, especially the part about beta carotene.)

In a similar vein, Kurt Butler, in his book *A Consumer's Guide to Alternative Medicine* (Prometheus, 1992), writes that lecithin "is alleged to lower cholesterol and to improve memory in normal and demented persons. There is some evidence for the first claim, but the effect is probably due to its polyunsaturated fat content, in which case it would be cheaper to simply consume more vegetable oil than to take lecithin. Definitive studies on this question have not been done." Butler concludes, "Unfortunately, there is no evidence to support the claim of improved memory in either normal persons or those with memory deficits." Actually, there have been several studies done in the area of memory. In a double-blind placebo-controlled trial of high-dose lecithin given to fifty-one patients with Alzheimer's disease, reported in 1985 in the *Journal of Neurology, Neurosurgery, and Psychiatry,* there were no differences between the placebo and the lecithin groups. More recently, in a study of fifty-three subjects with Alzheimer's disease reported in the *British Medical Journal* in 1994, lecithin was again found to have no better effect than a placebo.

❖ ❖ ❖   What's the bottom line on lecithin? There's no proof that it will do you any good. On the other hand, there is no risk in taking it, if you're so inclined. I do not prescribe it in my practice.

Well, the owner of my health food shop wants to close for the night, and my publisher won't give me any extra time to describe the multitude of other products on the shelves—all of which promise something for someone. Browse among them yourself, but before buying any, be sure to consult with your doctor. Remember that "natural" can be just as potent as "prescription."

INDEX

ABOUT THE AUTHOR

DR. ISADORE ROSENFELD is the Rossi Distinguished Professor of Clinical Medicine at New York Hospital–Cornell Medical Center. A longtime adviser to government on health matters, he recently completed four years of service as a member of the Practicing Physicians Advisory Council to the United States Secretary of Health and Human Services. He is also an overseer of Cornell University Medical College, a member of the Board of Visitors at the University of California School of Medicine at Davis, and on an advisory committee at the Emory University School of Medicine. Dr. Rosenfeld is a member of many major national and international medical organizations, including the American College of Cardiology, the American College of Physicians, the Royal College of Physicians (Canada), and the Royal Society of Medicine in Britain. He is a past president of the New York County Medical Society and was also chairman of its Board of Censors. He was the first recipient of the award for Achievement in Cardiovascular Medicine and Science by the New York affiliate of the American Heart Association. The Rosenfeld Heart Foundation, of which he is president, has for many years supported research in the area of cardiovascular disease here and abroad. Dr. Rosenfeld divides his time teaching, writing, and practicing medicine as a cardiologist in Manhattan. He and his wife, Camilla, live in Westchester County, New York. They have four children and two grandchildren.

ABOUT THE TYPE

This book was set in Century Schoolbook, a member of the Century family of typefaces. It was designed in the 1890s by Theodore Low DeVinne of the American Type Founders Company, in collaboration with Linn Boyd Benton. It was one of the earliest types designed for a specific purpose, the *Century* magazine, because it was able to maintain the economies of a narrower typeface while using stronger serifs and thickened verticals.